The Truth About Bodybuilding

A scientific approach

by

Stuart Cosgrove MCSP SRP

First published in Great Britain 2019

First edition 2019

ISBN: 978-1-792051-97-5

Copyright ©Stuart Cosgrove 2019

Tbb57

DEDICATION

This book is dedicated to all those people over the years who have either inspired or helped me in the accumulation of this knowledge. I will attempt to name some of the major influences and I apologise if I miss anybody out. Thanks go to Dorian Yates – six times Mr Olympia winner, Ernie Taylor – Top professional and high ranking Olympia contender. My most consistent training partners, namely John Donnellan, John Morgan, Phil Knight, Pat Lewarne and Brian Goddard who himself won various WABBA and EFBB national titles. Thanks to John Wardley, Patrick Higgins, Kerry Kayes, John Ramsey and Charlotte MacGill (Miss Universe 2014). Thanks also go to John Hodgson (we both sing from the same song sheet). Thanks to all these people for your help and support over the years. Finally, thanks to my lovely wife, Joanne, and my parents, Bill and Margaret, for their continued support.

Thanks also go to Tiago and Sandra Caldeira for filming and producing the DVD and also Chrissie Newby for help with the writing up and setting out.

FOREWORD
by Kerry Kayes

When I was asked to do a foreward by Stuart for his new book, I felt honoured and proud. I thought about all the people Stuart knows and has treated in his practice yet he has asked me, so I have taken this very seriously.

I first saw Stuart on a Sunday afternoon in a nightclub called Quaffers 30 years ago where he was competing in a UK Squatting competition. He had to squat 600lbs as many times as possible, whoever got the most reps won. Stuart won that day and it did not surprise me! I had heard of him from various gyms in the Bolton area as he was famous for bending bars whilst squatting! In fact Stuart had competed in a number of Strongman shows winning 3 of them and over 20 Bodybuilding shows.

Little did I know how important Stuart would become in my life. He is the best physio in the world in my opinion! I know this better than most as I have had most of the injuries in the book and Stuart has worked on all of them!

Dorian Yates, Ricky Hatton and many many more have relied on Stuart to get them through their training. In fact it is well documented that after working on Ricky's elbows he put another 2 inches on his reach! Something that is very important in the boxing ring!

One of my best memories was when Stuart and I were asked to go down to Temple Gym, Dorian's gym in Birmingham to see him 4 weeks before the 1993 Mr Olympia. It was an especially special moment because there was only Debbie (Dorian's wife), Dorian himself and Kevin Horton who was there to take those famous black and white photos, the ones where Dorian kept his socks on! Dorian looked probably the best he has ever looked in photos. It was a great moment and we were both there to witness it!

I've been all over the world with many sportsmen and Stuart was there to share some of my best memories. At the Mr Olympia contests in Long Beach and Las Vegas, Stuart treated Dorian in his room every hour through the night before the competitions to get him through the show, and the treatment clearly worked as Dorian won!

Stuart was also present in Las Vegas for some of Ricky's fights. The night before a fight, Stuart would 'click' Ricky's back and loosen him up for the fight. The next day, he would be in the dressing room in case anything went wrong.

Everybody knows that Ricky attracted some famous fans. One night Stuart was chatting to one of them. He asked Stuart "What do you do?". Stuart replied and said "I'm the physio to Ricky". Stuart then turned round and asked the stranger "So what do you do?". "I'm an actor" came back the reply. Stuart then turned round and said "I'm sorry but I didn't catch your name?" "Brad Pitt" came back the reply!!! I think that encounter sums up Stuart as he treats everybody the same. You can be one of the biggest stars or just a regular person and Stuart will be there for you!

Another thing about Stuart is that he also has more hobbies than anyone I know. Every year he goes to America Storm Chasing. He plays the guitar plus other instruments and produces his own instrumental guitar cd's. He has a massive interest in Roller Coasters and their history. He knows top designers of rides and has been included in the design of some of them. Believe me if anyone reading this book ever goes on 'Who Wants to be a Millionaire', I'd advise you to ask Stuart to be your 'Phone a Friend' !!

CONTENTS

Foreword
About the Author
Introduction

CHAPTERS

1 Muscle Structure and Function   Page 1
2 Energy Systems and Muscle Fibre Types   Page 17
3 How a Muscle Repairs and Grows   Page 31
4 Neural Adaptation to Weight Training   Page 46
5 Bodybuilding Methods through the Ages   Page 55
6 The Ideal Training Protocol for Muscle Growth   Page 76
7 Constructing a Training Program   Page 85
8 What Prevents a Muscle from Responding   Page 104
9 Common Injuries & Conditions affecting
   Bodybuilders   Page 124
10 Off-Season and Pre Contest Diet Plans   Page 151
11 Ergogenic Aids   Page 176
12 Healthy Bodybuilding for the Over 50's   Page 199
   Conclusions   Page 233
   References   Page 235

ABOUT THE AUTHOR

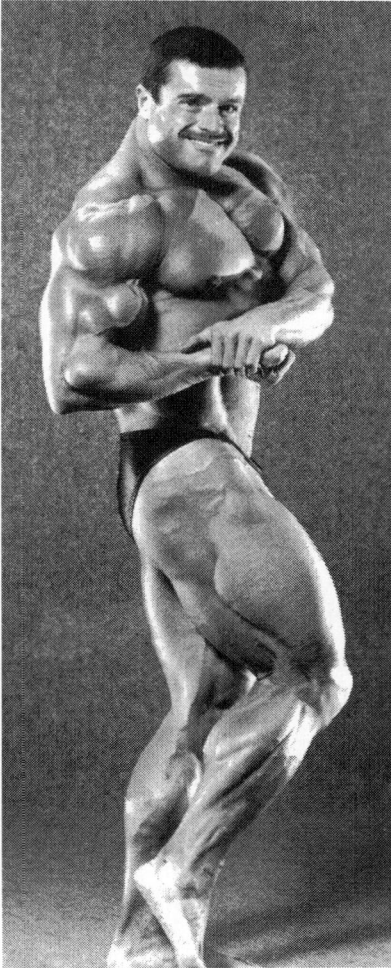

Stuart Cosgrove became interested in bodybuilding and physiotherapy about the same time back in 1976. He studied the various weight training principles of that time, eventually going on to study physiotherapy and qualifying from Salford University in 1982.

He studied post-graduation courses in acupuncture, sports injuries, strength and conditioning, myofascial techniques and manipulation. He started his private practice in 1987 and has successfully treated many world champions since, especially being involved in the careers of Dorian Yates for nine years, the boxer Ricky Hatton for eight years, and the bodybuilding champion Ernie Taylor for eight years. He has lectured on the master's degree course in strength and conditioning at Bolton University. He competed in bodybuilding competitions for 22 years from 1978 to 2000, winning various titles but mainly the NABBA Mr UK in 1987, the WABBA Mr Britain in 1996, and fourth place in the Mr Universe in 1992. He also won a number of power lifting/strongman competitions and became the UK's Squat Champion in 1989 with 600lbs for twelve repetitions.

He always has and continues to be interested in the practical applications of muscle physiology with regard to the development of muscle.

INTRODUCTION

Even from the times of Milo, the five time Olympic Games winner in ancient Greece over 2,000 years ago, people have explored progressive resistance training to develop the physique both for visual cosmetic benefits and also for the physical benefits. Over time, many weight training systems have been employed, some have been closely linked to one another, some based on sound physiological backing and others based around pure myth. Ever since the 1930s the bodybuilding scene has been like the fashion industry, coming round in circles, fads coming and going, many of them not based on true physiology but based on a particular personality trying to push a particular style of training in vogue at the time.

Right up to today, the bodybuilding fraternity is littered with self-professing gurus who latch on to a particular principle, sometimes without really analysing whether or not it stands up under scientific scrutiny. What this book is designed to do is examine what it takes to make a muscle grow and adapt, examining the scientific principles and then finding the best training principle incorporating these ideas in a practical way.

We will examine many of the more tried and tested bodybuilding principles over the last few decades and then we will see if they stand up to scientific scrutiny and take the best of each system in order to devise the best possible complete training system to apply to develop muscles as fully as possible.

As you go through this book you will see at the end of each chapter there is an abstract section which is, basically, a brief summary of an in-depth analysis of the particular subject dealt with in that chapter. It is designed for those people who want to understand as much as possible the scientific basis for these training techniques but are not willing to look too in-depth at the deep scientific research. It gives people a take home message or conclusion of the subject the chapter covers.

CHAPTER 1
MUSCLE STRUCTURE AND FUNCTION

Physical exercise and sports performance involves effective and purposeful movements of the body. These movements result from the forces developed in muscles. These muscles, acting through lever systems of the skeleton, move the various body parts. Skeletal muscles are under the control of the cerebral cortex in the brain which works through nerve fibres or motor neurons to activate these skeletal muscles. Contracting the muscle fibres pulls against the tendon, which then pulls against the bone that it's attached to, which then moves that bone over its respective joint. Support for this neuromuscular activity involves continuous delivery of energy systems, involving oxygen too, and removal of carbon dioxide from working tissues through the activities of the cardiovascular and the respiratory system.

The interaction of all these systems is important to understand for the strength and conditioning professional. We will not go into too much detail about the microscopic structure of muscle tissue as it is unnecessary for our needs at this time. However, a general overview of the muscular system and how it functions, combined with the nerve system that supplies it is essential in order to prescribe the best exercise protocols for improving the muscle, both in strength and power.

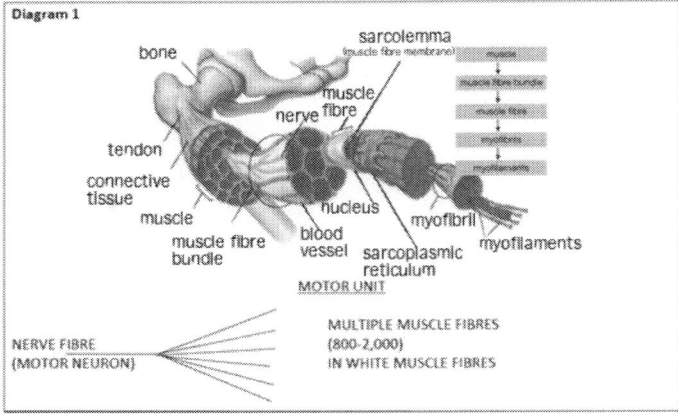

Diagram 1

bone
sarcolemma (muscle fibre membrane)
muscle fibre
nerve
tendon
connective tissue
muscle
muscle fibre bundle
nucleus
blood vessel
myofibril
sarcoplasmic reticulum
myofilaments

muscle
muscle fibre bundle
muscle fibre
myofibres
myofilaments

MOTOR UNIT

NERVE FIBRE (MOTOR NEURON)

MULTIPLE MUSCLE FIBRES (800-2,000) IN WHITE MUSCLE FIBRES

Diagram 2

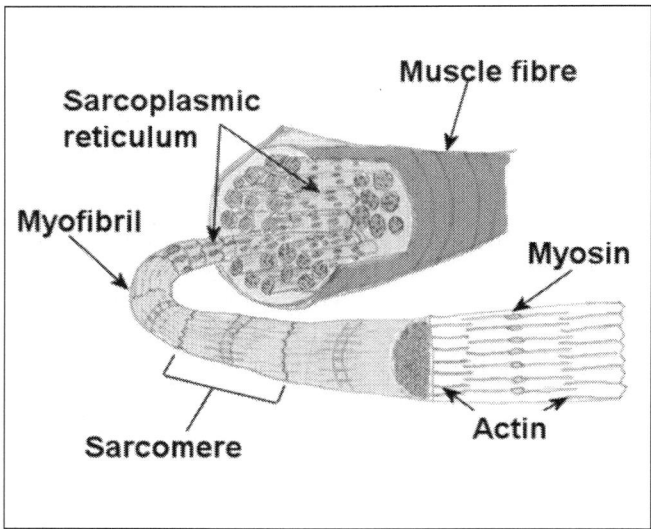

Sarcoplasmic reticulum

Muscle fibre

Myofibril

Myosin

Sarcomere

Actin

2

As we look at diagrams 1 and 2, we see that the muscle is initially attached to the bone via a tendon. The tendon connective tissue is very strong and inelastic and provides a firm anchor for the muscle to initiate movement on the bone. The opposite end of the muscle is attached, again, by a tendon over a joint to an associated bone in order to provide movement by contraction. As you can see, the overall structure of the muscle starts off with a connective tissue on the outside of it. This connective tissue is known as fascia. This fascia interacts with adjoining muscles and also envelops the tendons as well. It interacts with all the connective tissues throughout the body.

We'll go on to discover how important this thin inelastic fascial tissue is when we consider how it's needed to keep the muscular system working efficiently. As we go down almost to microscopic level through the muscle, we notice that the muscle fibres are constructed in bundles and they eventually come down into smaller myofibril filaments. Inside these myofibril filaments are two proteins called Myosin and Actin. These two proteins form cross ridges which attach to one another and draw the two proteins closer together. This then acts as a contraction of the muscle, and the muscle ends up in a shortened state. This provides the movement of the bones over the joint.

If we go back to diagram 1 you'll notice another small diagram there of a motor unit. A motor unit is composed of a nerve fibre, or motor neuron, which connects to multiple muscle fibres. As we'll go on to see, when we talk about muscle fibre types, the type of muscle that produces strong explosive contractions are called Fast Twitch fibres, or white muscle fibres. Each nerve fibre that's attached to these white fibres can connect to as many as 800 to 2,000 fibres. So that's one nerve fibre connecting to 800 to 2,000 muscle fibres. Each of these motor units contracts in an all-or-none fashion. In other words, if the motor nerve is excited, or the nerve fibre excited, it will stimulate all of the muscle fibres to contract. That is, all of the muscle fibres within that particular motor unit.

As you can imagine, larger motor units, i.e. those nerve fibres that connect to many muscle fibres generate more tension because they're composed of more muscle fibres. As they contract, the strength of the contraction is much larger. Generally speaking, larger muscles responsible for larger movements contain larger motor units. For example, our bicep muscle is a relatively large muscle and is responsible for relatively large movements. Its motor units are quite large, with a single motor neuron or nerve fibre innervating thousands of muscle fibres. Eye muscles, on the other hand, generate small contractions and thus small movements of the eyes. So these muscles contain very small motor units, and each nerve fibre may only supply as little as ten muscle fibres. As you increase the stimulus to the muscle by adding weight, or resistance to that muscle contraction, you will recruit, gradually, more and more motor units until the muscle has no more available to activate. This is classed as a maximum contraction. As you warm up the muscle, adding more weight slowly, you will recruit more motor units.

Later on, in Chapter 5, when we talk about the ideal training protocol for muscle growth, we will talk about performing a primer set just before you perform the working set. This primer set will be almost maximum resistance. When you perform this primer set, which is close to your maximum weight, you fire up as many motor units as you can do. So the muscle works almost maximally but for a short time. Because you only do this one or two times, you don't use up all the energy in the muscle. You do, however, retain a motor memory for these motor units that have been contracted. When you then come to perform your working set with your maximum weight, all these motor units fire up simultaneously straight away. This allows the weight to move much more efficiently and a maximum stimulus is achieved to the muscle. In the DVD associated with this book, you will see me demonstrate a levitation trick, which isn't really a trick, and it demonstrates how effective performing of this primer set before your working set is.

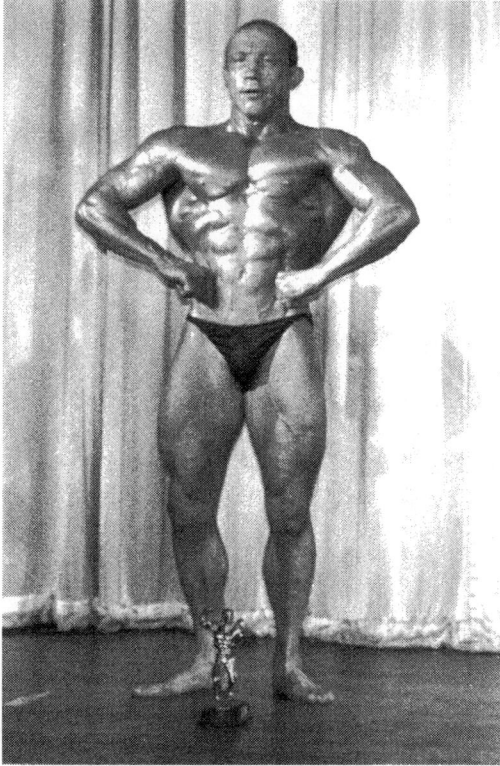

Pat Lewarne: Along with Brian Goddard and John Donnellan , my most loyal training partner, who took everything I threw at him and still came back for more! He achieved this condition winning the MR Manchester Over 40's.

Muscles and Fascia

Have you ever tried to watch a movie from the front row? Difficult, isn't it? Miserable as well. Very often the practice of medicine is such that medical text books tend to overemphasise the taking apart of the human body, dividing it, subdividing it and dividing it some more. It tends to give student doctors a "front row" perspective of anatomy and physiology. If you think about it, we have specialists in many fields, heart specialists, bone specialists, stomach specialists, arthritis specialists, mental health specialists. Unfortunately, this model can sometimes seem out of date. It fails miserably as far as really advancing our understanding of the human body because, really, you never get to see the big picture. It cannot explain how the whole body is greater than the sum of its individual parts.

5

Consider this example; Hydrogen, an explosive gas, plus oxygen, a flammable gas, gives you water, H_2O, a liquid, the foundation of life, and that's used to quench fire!! The problem with using outdated models that subdivide the body into increasingly smaller parts is that the big picture is frequently missed. Doctors use this same type of thought process when trying to explain the musculoskeletal system. When you look at the fascia in regard to the musculoskeletal system, it's one of the best examples of this. Doctors frequently miss the woods for the trees. Doctors are trained in the same kind of reductionist philosophy, they often use anatomical books that show hundreds of pictures of hundreds of individual muscles, without ever really showing or explaining the fascia. A chap called Henry Gray, probably the greatest illustrator of anatomy, wrote a text book over 150 years ago that is still considered to be one of the greatest anatomical books out there, and in many of his illustrations he left the fascia intact. So now we've spoken about the fascia, let us explain what it really is.

What is Fascia?

Fascia is a tough layer of fibrous collagen type connective tissue that permeates the whole body. If you hunt, very often you find people who hunt calling this silver skin, striffin. It's like a white, cellophane-like sack membrane that envelopes tightly around the muscles. Fascia surrounds individual muscles, muscle bundles, it's within individual muscles, groups of muscles, blood vessels and nerves. It binds these structures together in much the same manner that a plastic wrap is used to hold the contents of food together. Fascia consists of several extremely thin layers and is the tissue where the musculoskeletal system, circulatory system and nervous system all converge. It extends from the top of the head to the tip of the toes. Like ligaments and tendons, it's closely packed with bundles of wavy collagen fibres that line up in an organised and parallel fashion. The fascia supports and contains all these structures and is able to resist great tensile forces.

6

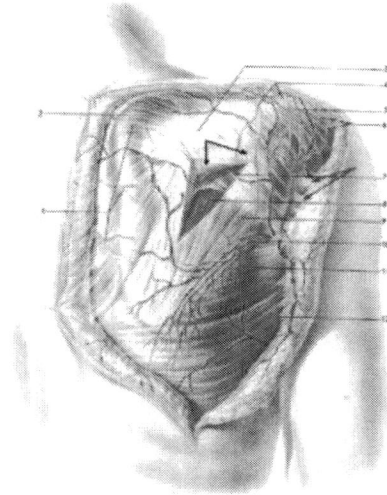

All arrows point to Fascia

Critical Functions of Healthy Fascia

1. It binds and holds muscles together compactly.
2. It ensures proper alignment of muscle fibres, blood vessels, nerves and other tissues within the muscle itself.
3. It transmits forces and loads evenly throughout the entire muscle.
4. It creates a uniformly smooth surface that essentially lubricates the various surfaces that come into contact with it during movement.
5. It allows the muscle to change shape as it lengthens or shortens.

Muscles are too often given the blame for a lot of musculoskeletal conditions and yet, by design, they cannot be involved in causing too many problems. They are often forced into doing things that they are not able to do. Muscles are often victims of circumstance and should be treated with care and respect. They are not only the slave units of the nervous system, but are also very dependent on the blood flow and their space supplied by the fascia for their function. If all these factors are present and working well, then the muscle will function as normal. However, if any one of these three factors is in a state of dysfunction, then the muscle simply will not work 100 percent.

7

There are three basic properties to muscle that will affect its function, there are:
1. Muscle is made up of elastic fibres.
2. Muscles have a vast blood supply.
3. Muscles have a poor sensory nerve supply.

Compare this with the main properties of fascia, namely:
1. Fascia is made up of mainly inelastic fibres.
2. Fascia has a very poor natural blood supply.
3. Fascia has a very rich sensory nerve supply.

As we can see, fascia, by being inelastic, has less give than muscle, and it will be damaged or strained first so as to protect the muscle. This is also why it has a poor natural blood supply as it does tear often during a normal day's activity, but cannot afford to bleed too heavily every time there is a tear.

Fascia is the protector not only of muscles but of all tissues and organs. The fascia, consisting of the pericardium for example, protects the heart. It also prevents it from over-expanding during the filling phase. At the same time it is acting as a resistance for the heart muscles to rebound against, to get greater force with which to push the blood out into the aorta. Fascia is an adaptable container with multidirectional fibres, and thus it is able to mould itself around different structures and adapt its shape as the structure changes. So, for example, if a muscle contracts, the fascia will close its cross fibres and take up the shape of the muscle, releasing when the muscle relaxes. The trouble starts when the fascia becomes dehydrated, either through overuse or if its blood supply is diminished and the fibres begin to shrink. The fascia is so reliant on its water content for functioning maximally. Also, whenever a muscle is overused or injured, doing heavy repetitive lifts or a repetitive job, over time collagen microfibers form in between adjacent layers of fascia and also the surface of the tissue that the fascia's supporting to bind them together so that the muscles can heal. These microfibers are sort of like nature's internal cast. Now, unfortunately, these casts do not automatically go away after the area has healed, and they tend to accumulate over time.

If something causes a fascia to exceed its normal tensile capacity, there will be a disruption or a micro-tearing of individual collagen fibres and this, in turn, leads to fascial scarring and adhesions. So if you combine this with the dehydrated fascia, you have a really tight container of the muscle that is sticking to other fascial containers close by and this, obviously, affects the function of the muscle. Once the fascia is injured, the microscopic fibres become disrupted and deranged. So instead of fibres running parallel to each other in an organised fashion with their normal degree of flexibility, the fibres now run in every possible direction in all three dimensions and have extremely diminished amount of organisation and elasticity.

If you take this concept of fascial shrinkage into muscle building, in a case where there's been a muscle wasting, say, for example, being bound up in a Plaster of Paris for a while, it is not just the muscle that suffers but also the fascia. The fascia will shrink to as to adapt to the new shape of the muscle. If the muscle is to be strengthened it will be imperative that the fascia becomes as mobile as possible, otherwise the muscle will not have the space in which to build, thus restricting muscle growth. Fascial shrinkage will also bring about postural changes as the body gives in to the tension of the fascia, thus changing its shape. Trying to correct posture against the inelastic pull without correcting the fascial tension will only result in more irritation and thus further adaptation.

So with the information we now have we can see that the flexibility of the human body is not governed just by the muscles which are elastic, but by the inelastic fibres of the fascia and other connective tissues. Good function depends on good muscle action. Good muscle action depends on flexible and hydrated fascia. Flexible, hydrated fascia depends on good blood flow. Stiffness, in the majority of cases, is not muscle or joint related but fascia related.

Thus, treatment should be aimed at the fascia initially. I would like to bring in the word posture here, as it is an interesting term that I think has been overused and misunderstood. Mention the

9

word posture to a layperson and it conjures up thoughts of being upright, rigid, a stationary position, shoulders back, chin up. However, posture is all about movement, not something that is static. The body is never static, but always in a state of flux. Posture follows movement like a shadow. Every tiny movement that takes place in the body brings about a new posture. It will, thus, be true to say that any changes in the shape and structure of the fascia will lead to a new posture. Take, for example, someone who works at a computer all day and does not have a good ergonomic setup. There is a tendency to slump and protrude the chin to compensate. This allows shortening of the posterior fascia of the neck, and this then will change the way that a person carries their head. If physiotherapists tell that person to correct their posture by straightening their neck, it would be going against the inelastic tendency of the fascia and cause more stress on it. However, if we release that fascia manually and restore its integrity, and also ensure its blood supply is back to normal, then the posture will restore itself. If the fascia is not mobile, then our POSTURE cannot be correct.

The Autonomic Nervous System (ANS)

This is the life of the body, it is the controller of all function as it is the controller of blood flow rate in the body. It, in turn, is dependent on the thyroid that has an organic control over the ANS, but it also needs blood flow. So there is a symbiotic setup in the body where one system needs the next and vice versa. I will not go into great depths about the anatomy of the ANS as it is extensive and these details can be found in appropriate books. The part of the ANS that we will need to discuss is called the Sympathetic Nervous System or the SNS. The SNS runs in two chains of nerve cells parallel to the spine under the angle of the ribcage. They have been so placed compared to within the spine so as not to be jeopardised when the spine is damaged. They thus have more freedom to move and resist stress that can be susceptible to certain stresses such as shock and overload. They are severely stressed by whiplash injuries and direct trauma to the back and an explosive trauma to the spine, as in gunshots to the back.

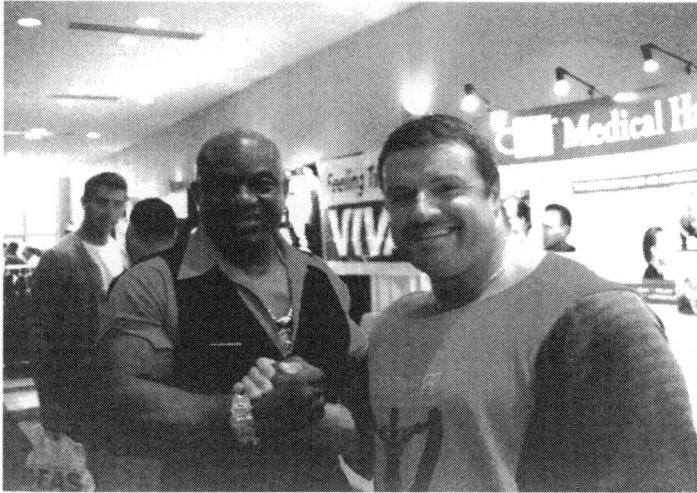

Sergio Oliva: Here we are chatting about training during the 1995 Mr Olympia when all the past winners were present on stage together.

The main function of the SNS is to control the tone of the blood vessels. The nerves piggyback on the blood vessels and fire off in a fashion that causes a peristaltic like action or a squeezing effect to occur on the vessel walls. This action is effective in squeezing the blood in the vessels from the heart to the rest of the body. There is a fundamental rate at which this occurs and it is variable at different times of the day. During the day, the SNS is very active and there is more demand for blood, but as the body begins to rest and then sleep this system will slow down so as to allow the brain and body to sleep. If we look at the table on stress response you will see that if the demand on the SNS is too much it will reach a state of fatigue whereby it will initially decrease in activity, and then it will switch into an emergency mode and begin firing at a higher than

11

normal rate. This will happen for a while and then it will fatigue further and eventually lose control of what it is meant to do. This will lead to a relaxing of arterial tone and, thus, a slowing of the blood flow rate. Because it controls its own blood flow, the SNS will obviously starve itself of blood flow in this state and it will set up a vicious cycle of events which will deteriorate rapidly.

The 'Stress Response'

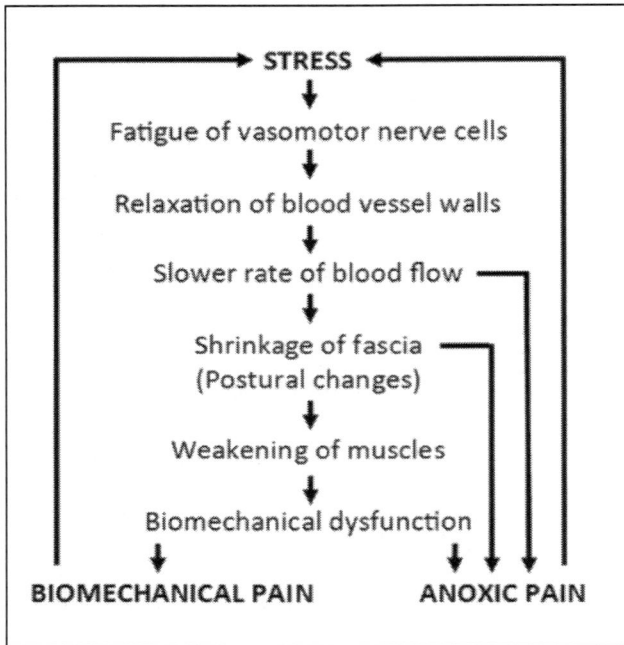

As you can see from the stress response table, our bodies have a certain pattern that they keep to when put under enough stress so as to go beyond the limits of control. The stress can be physical, mental, energetic or emotional, or a combination of all four. If it goes beyond the body's threshold then it will begin to cause damage to the body. The body has a fantastic ability to compensate, but once the limits are breached it will be exposed and will begin to wear. Changes take place initially on an energetic basis, and then physiological, and then physical.

Mental and emotional symptoms may also result from this. One thing we need to be aware of here is that stress itself is not the problem. It is the body's inability to deal with stress that must be addressed.

One of the most common complaints that we are confronted with is repetitive strain injury, or repetitive stress injury (RSI). If we take a closer look at most of the complaints we see we could probably say that approximately 85 percent are some form of RSI. The tendency is to think of RSI as being a result of physical activity, yet sitting on a chair for hours on end can be a form of RSI as some tissues are being held in a fixed tone for lengthy periods of time, which in its own right is a form of overload. Take a computer operator for example. To allow for fine work to be done with the hands, the shoulder girdle must be fixed in a stable position. This now makes a demand on the shoulder girdle muscles which are designed predominantly for movement (unlike postural muscles) to remain in a semi-fixed tone for long periods. For this to be able to occur, the vasomotor nerve cells of the SNS controlling the blood flow to this area have to work extra hard to deliver the necessary blood to these muscles. This causes overload of the nerve cells and, thus, an alteration in the blood flow to the muscles from a relaxation of the vascular tone. This leads to fatigue of the muscles, shrinkage of the fascia in the area and a build-up of ischemic or anoxic pain (see the diagram). Therefore, we can see that RSI is not a result of strain on the muscles and soft tissues but a strain on the sympathetic nervous system or the SNS. Treatment for the majority of conditions we see should, therefore, effectively begin by improving circulatory supply.

In fact, I would go as far as to say that nearly all conditions should be treated as if they are circulatory conditions primarily. The Chinese have been saying this for thousands of years, where there is pain there is blood stagnation or congestion, often using acupuncture to alleviate this. As a result of this, it is apparent that rest is not always the answer in treatment of these conditions. If you refer to the DVD accompanying this book, you will see various techniques demonstrated.

13

If we start, firstly, by trying to improve circulatory stagnation, we use various techniques, one being acupuncture, another one is myofascial release techniques. We use manipulation to prevent adhesion formation in joints and we also see demonstrated the Cryoflow technique, which is a means by which we stimulate these vasomotor nerve cells in the SNS into activity again, reenergising them and providing more blood supply to the muscles concerned. A lot of you reading this and going through this section will be thinking, "What's this got to do with bodybuilding?" Well, in short, a lot. If you think about it, every time you train intensely with heavy resistance you're causing not only damage to the muscle tissue itself, but also micro tear damage to the fascia, which can then result in a lot of the factors that we've discussed in this chapter. So it's so important for the bodybuilder to stay on top of all these conditions that can occur which can affect blood flow to the muscle and, therefore, obviously it can affect performance and hypertrophy.

I always recommend bodybuilders to incorporate within their timetable physiotherapy treatment techniques such as myofascial release, acupuncture, manipulation and maintain flexibility of the musculoskeletal system as well in order to maximise performance. Further guidelines on treatment and regularity of treatment will be given in Chapter 9 of this book.

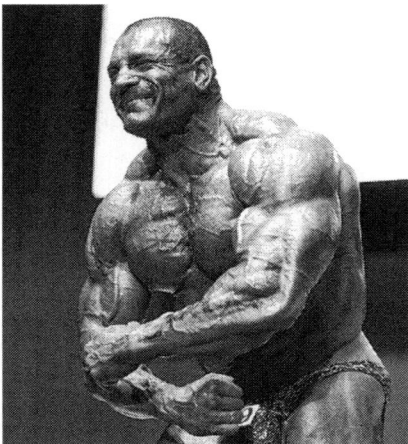

Martin Stephenson: Martin took his physique to another level utilising these training principles in this book, culminating in a NABBA Mr Universe win! I was proud to help him achieve his goal!

Chapter 1 - Muscle Structure and Function Summary

1. The cerebral cortex initiates muscle contraction through nerve fibres.
2. Myosin and Actin filaments interact in the muscle to contract it.
3. A motor unit comprises of a nerve fibre attached to multiple muscle fibres.
4. Motor units work on the principle of the all-or-nothing rule. They are either switched on or off, contracting all their respective muscle fibres or not.
5. Motor unit memory, once they're maximal (or close to maximal) contraction is achieved, the neuromuscular system remembers this response for up to five minutes and this motor summation contraction can be called upon instantly again within this time, leading to more productive working sets (see Chapter 5).
6. Fascia is a tough fibrous connective tissue layer that encompasses muscles and organs and permeates the whole body.
7. Fascia has;
    a) a relatively poor flexibility
    b) a poor blood supply
    c) good sensory nerve supply
8. Muscles have;
    a) good flexibility
    b) good blood supply
    c) poor sensory nerve supply
9. Fascia adapts its shape to conform to the muscle shape.
10. Fascia tears repeatedly during heavy activities more than the muscle does.
11. Fascial damage may lead to adhesions and cause the muscle to dysfunction.
12. Posture is affected by tight adhesed fascia.
13. The ANS (the Autonomic Nervous System) consists of the Sympathetic (SNS) and Parasympathetic (PNS) systems. These two systems work in conjunction with one another but we will be concerned mainly with the SNS.

15

14. <u>The SNS</u>. This is the Sympathetic Nervous System and consists of chains of nerve cells running inside the ribcage. These supply nerve fibres to control muscle blood vessels, supplying blood to muscles, other nerves and other tissues.
15. <u>Overload of SNS</u> can lead to blood supply reduction, ischaemia (loss of circulation and oxygen) of muscles and, therefore, postural dysfunction and injury.
16. <u>Treatment techniques</u> to prevent or relieve this situation are acupuncture, myofascial release, manipulation and Cryoflow techniques (see Chapter 9).

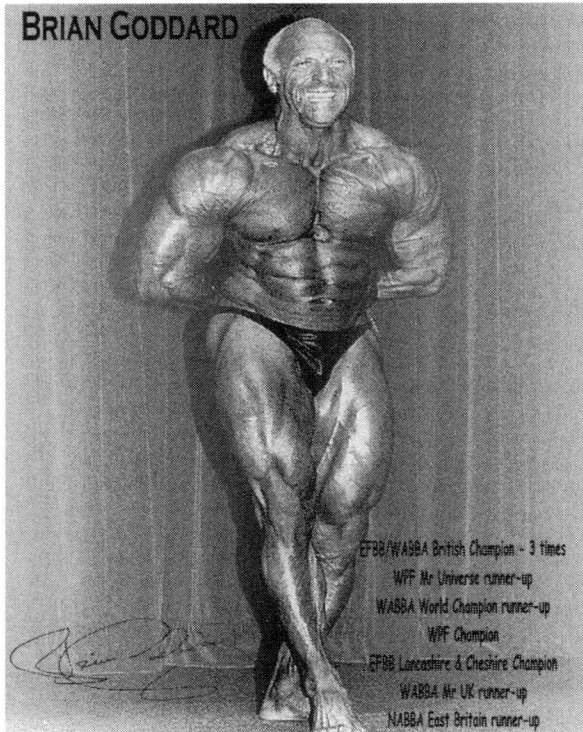

BRIAN GODDARD

EFBB/WABBA British Champion - 3 times
WPF Mr Universe runner-up
WABBA World Champion runner-up
WPF Champion
EFBB Lancashire & Cheshire Champion
WABBA Mr UK runner-up
NABBA East Britain runner-up

Brian Goddard: Winner of mutiple Senior EFBB British Titles. My training partner for 20+ years.

16

CHAPTER 2.
Energy Systems and Muscle Fibre Types

Energy Systems

Our own bodies, like all living organisms, are energy conversion machines. Conversion of energy implies that the chemical energy stored in food is converted into work, thermal energy, or is stored in fatty tissue as chemical energy (see Diagram 3a). By far the largest portion of this energy ingested in food goes to thermal energy, although this portion varies depending on the type of physical activity done. The portion going into each form depends on how much we eat and on our level of physical activity. If we eat more than is needed to work and stay warm, the remainder goes into body fat. So we can see that the fat reserves are really like an overflow or a storage depot of energy.

Diagram 3a

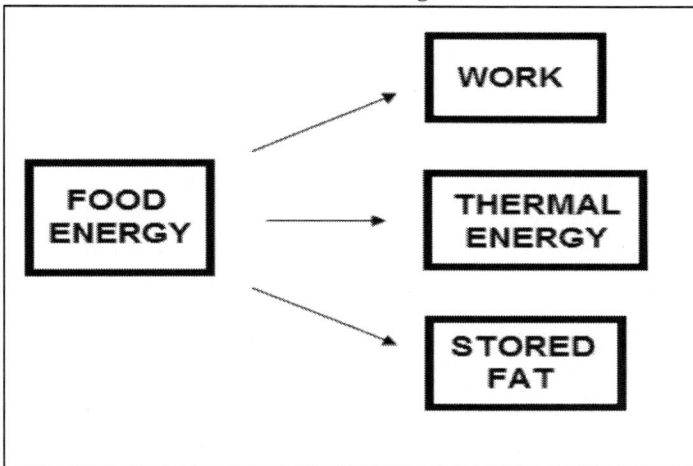

All bodily functions, from thinking to lifting weights, require energy. The many small muscle actions accompanying all quiet activity, from sleeping to head scratching, ultimately become thermal energy, as do less visible muscle actions by the heart and the lungs, and the digestive tract. In fact, shivering, which is an involuntary response to low body temperature, pits muscles against one another to produce thermal energy in the body so the muscle work actually converts to thermal energy. The kidneys and the liver consume a surprising amount of energy, but the biggest surprise of all is that a full 25 percent of all energy consumed by the body is used to maintain the brain and the nervous system. Electrical impulses darting around through nerves and tiny impulses in the brain use up a phenomenal amount of energy. This bioelectrical energy ultimately also becomes thermal energy but some is utilised to power chemical processes such as in the kidney and the liver, and also in fat production.

Basal Metabolic Rate (BMR)

The rate at which the body uses food energy to sustain life and to do different activities is called the metabolic rate. The total energy conversion rate of a person at rest is called the Basal Metabolic Rate and is divided among the various systems in the body. So this is the amount of energy that is required just to sustain the body at rest. Because muscle uses a greater amount of energy than other tissues, such as fat, the BMR for athletes is usually greater for this reason. Efficient and productive training programmes can be designed through an understanding of how energy is made available for specific types of exercise and how energy transfer can be modified by specific training regimes.

Before we start looking at energy systems in more detail, we need to establish some terminology used. If we start off by defining energy as the ability or capacity to perform work, it is the breakdown of the chemical bonds in food that provides the energy necessary to perform biological work. This breakdown of larger molecules into smaller ones associated with the release of energy is called catabolism. So these reactions are catabolic and generally involve an energy release. Conversely, the synthesis of larger molecules from smaller molecules can be accomplished using the energy released from these catabolic reactions, and this building up process is termed anabolism.

So if we think about the breakdown of proteins into amino acids, this is an example of catabolism, whilst the formation of proteins from amino acids in cells, specifically muscle cells, is an anabolic process.

The energy derived from catabolic reactions is used to drive anabolic reactions through an intermediate molecule called ATP. So if we think of ATP (Adenosine Triphosphate) as the chemical that allows the transfer of energy into an anabolic response, we can see that without an adequate supply of ATP, muscular activity and muscle growth would not be possible. This is apparent when designing training programmes for strength and conditioning. When an ATP molecule breaks down to yield energy, this is known as hydrolysis because it requires water to do this. So the hydrolysis of ATP results in biological work. This is an anabolic response and can be used to produce energy to contract a muscle or to synthesise new proteins into cells.

Diagram 3b

Aerobic:	Using Oxygen
Anaerobic:	Without Using Oxygen
Lactic:	Forming Lactate
Alactic:	Without Forming Lactate

ENERGY SYSTEM	SUBSTRATE	DURATION OF EXERCISE	BREAKDOWN	AVAILABILITY	SPEED OF ENERGY PRODUCTION
A	Creating Phosphate (Cp)	0 – 10 secs	Anaerobic Alactic	Very Limited	Very Fast
B	Glycogen or	10 – 30 secs	Anaerobic Lactic	Limited	Fast
	Glucose	30 sec – 3 min	Aerobic Lactic		
C	Glycogen or Glucose	3 mins – few hours	Aerobic Alactic	Limited	Slow
D	Fatty Acids	10 mins – unlimited	Aerobic Alactic	Unlimited	Sluggish

Systems C and D begin to work together from 10 minutes onwards with energy from fats gradually increasing.

We will consider four types of energy system. As you can see from Diagram 3b, I've listed those systems as A, B, C and D.

19

We will go through each system in turn but as an overview you can see that starting off at A, depending on the duration and intensity of the exercise, we can see that A is the first line of defence or the first energy producing system, and D is the last, or the slowest energy producing system. After ten minutes, all four energy systems are interrelated and work to different degrees in supplying energy for muscle work. Energy system A is usually classed as the Creatine Phosphate or the phosphagen energy system. Energy systems B and C are classed as glycolysis.

Glycolysis is the breakdown of carbohydrates either from carbohydrates stored in the muscles as glycogen, or glucose delivered in the blood to produce ATP for energy. Some of the energy systems are classed as aerobic, which means utilising oxygen, and some are classed as anaerobic which can continue without using oxygen. Some are lactic and some are alactic. This means some form lactate and some don't form lactate, and we will explain this shortly.

Getting back to energy system A, this is the phosphagen system, so Creatine Phosphate produces (when it breaks down) ATP to supply energy and Creatine. Creatine Phosphate is stored in the muscle and usually the larger the muscle, the more Creatine Phosphate you can store. This can also be supplemented, but it needs to be noted that excess Creatine that's produced from this reaction can be reconverted back into Creatine Phosphate again.

It's worth bearing in mind that it takes about three minutes to reenergise the Creatine Phosphate system to more than 50 percent and approximately eight minutes to reach hundred percent levels again. Although Creatine Phosphate is utilised in very explosive intense exercise, it is also used up gradually throughout the day in normal metabolism. Helping to replenish this in supplement form can sometimes help to make sure that the system is charged a hundred percent prior to intense exercise.

As you can see from the diagram, the Creatine Phosphate is only used for the first ten seconds then it gets very depleted if the exercise is intense enough. It produces a very fast energy response and is utilised by Type II or white muscle fibres. Its breakdown doesn't require oxygen, and it doesn't produce lactate in the muscle as a bi-product. So this is a very useful energy source for lifting heavy weights maximally. As it is constantly replenished throughout long endurance activities, it's also a useful substrate for sprints at the end of a long endurance race.

During intense exercise from ten seconds onwards, the main energy system utilised is B. If we look at B, it's split up into two types of glycolysis. The first type lasts up to 30 seconds and doesn't require oxygen. However, it does produce lactate. When we look at the first type of glycolysis in energy system B, the one that lasts up to 30 seconds, when the glycogen or glucose breaks down to produce ATP for energy, it also produces pyruvate. This pyruvate then converts to lactate, and the lactate that builds up in the muscle can be resynthesized back into ATP again. So this can be cleared from the muscle and transported into the blood and oxidised, or it can be transported in the blood back to the liver where it's converted back to glucose.

The second half of energy system B, where the glucose is broken down with oxygen present, it still forms lactic acid, but then the pyruvate that is produced then gets incorporated back into the cell without producing lactate, and the mitochondria of the cell resynthesize ATP using a cycle called Krebs cycle. As this continues on we move into energy system C, which is aerobic, but it doesn't produce lactate in the muscle because the pyruvate is completely taken up by the mitochondria in the cells.

To summarise this, if the exercise is very intense, then the first part of energy system B will come into play, producing a lot of lactate in the muscle. If the exercise intensity decreases you move into energy system C which utilises oxygen, and this can be continued for a few hours. This is limited by the amount of glycogen stored in the muscles, or glucose in the bloodstream.

The final energy system, energy system D, is the utilisation of fatty acids. Fats can be oxidised for energy from triglycerides stored in fat cells, can be broken down into free fatty acids which go into the bloodstream where they circulate and enter muscle fibres. These can then be oxidised to produce ATP. This, again, enters the Krebs cycle to produce the energy. Because this system is very slow, the energy production is very slow. So where energy requirements are less, either if you're resting at a computer desk or you're just resting on the couch, you will be mainly burning fatty acids for energy. Also, if you switch from a very high intensity exercise to a low intensity exercise the highest proportion of the energy production will come from fatty acids. This is useful to know when doing fat burning to try and improve condition as an athlete, that if you keep your intensity level down low, say, on an exercise cycle, you can burn more fat than carbohydrate. Energy system D is unlimited, so it could be from ten minutes to an unlimited period because you're utilising your fat storage.

In a similar way to energy system D, although we've not listed it here as a primary energy producer, it must be noted that proteins can be utilised also as energy. Proteins are utilised for energy production in three situations;

1) If the protein ingestion in the diet is excessive but more than what is required for the synthesis of new proteins in cells, then the excess protein can be oxidised for energy. The protein can be broken down into its constituent amino acids and then converted into glucose in a process known as gluconeogenesis. This produces ATP for energy.

2) If the exercise is of long enough duration and high enough intensity that carbohydrate levels are depleted somewhat, then protein breakdown can occur, either utilisation of ingested protein or breakdown of cellular protein from muscle can occur to produce energy.

3) If not enough carbohydrates are ingested in the diet to sustain energy levels for muscular activity. If the glycogen levels are depleted too much in the muscles then protein break down from either ingested protein or cellular protein can occur. The contribution of amino acids to the production of ATP energy has been

22

estimated to be anything from three to 18 percent of the energy requirement during a prolonged activity if carbohydrate levels are depleted.

It must be noted here that most of the oxidation coming from protein is from the branched chain amino acids in the muscle. A lot of research has been done to suggest that maintaining levels of branched chain amino acids in the muscle during activity or immediately post-activity can help to offset muscle degradation.

If we think how we can apply the knowledge we've learnt here in constructing our programme, we can see that the energy system A produces a massive energy production for the first ten seconds followed by energy system B. As we go on to discuss about muscle fibre types we'll see that the maximum time under tension we want to sustain the muscle ideally is within the time constraints of energy systems A and B. The two main problems that we come up against are the breakdown of Creatine Phosphate very quickly and also the production of lactate in the muscle from energy system B. As we've already learnt, Creatine could be rephosphorylised into Creatine Phosphate again. This process takes approximately three minutes to achieve 50 percent of its capacity. The hydrolysis of ATP in the Creatine system causes hydrogen ions and Phosphate levels to rise in the muscle.

Increasing Phosphate levels reduces the cross ridge formation for muscle contraction so the muscle is not able to contract the same. Also the hydrogen ions produced from the hydrolysis of ATP combined with the lactate which increased the acidosis in the muscle inhibits the nerve muscle connection, thereby also reducing muscle contraction. Both the removal of the Phosphate and the hydrogen ions from both these systems takes approximately three minutes. As we've already learned, it takes about three minutes to reenergise the CP system back to 50 percent. It is logical to assume, based on this knowledge, that a longer rest time in between sets is required. After the final warm up, or primer set, before a working set, this needs to be taken into consideration. Most people when they train, especially if they train on their own, tend not to rest long enough in between sets and, therefore, these systems are affected, which leads to either muscle inhibition or a lack of maximal, forceful contraction of the muscle and, therefore, a less productive set.

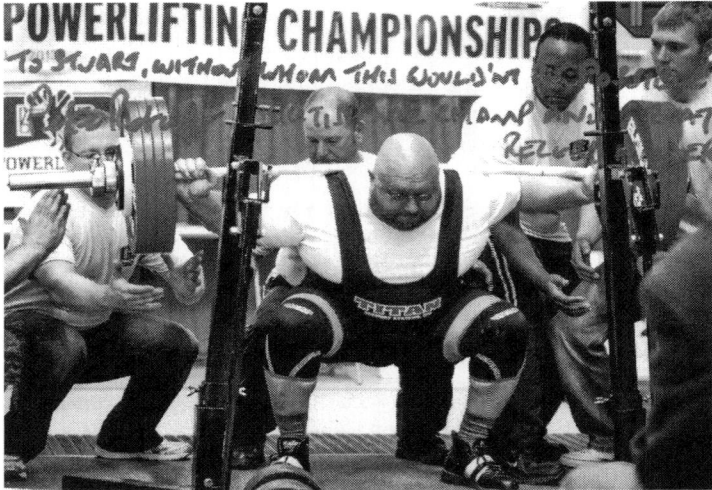

Peter Ratcliffe: A senior multiple Powerlifting record holder, who applied some of these bodybuilding principles into his training.

Muscle Fibre Types

It's so important when devising bodybuilding programmes that we look at muscle fibre types. Very often when people come up to me and ask me for a programme, and I start to describe the programme which would be most productive for muscle and strength gains, they usually reply, "Oh, well, that doesn't apply to me, I've got a different muscle fibre type that responds differently to training." Whilst it must be said that we all vary slightly genetically, some people have a predisposition to a different type of muscle fibre, it must be said that we are all from the same planet, with the same physiology and we respond to the same muscle overload. The only difference is that there will be a variation in the response. If two people are given the

24

same exercise programme there will be a difference in results obtained. However, one thing can be guaranteed, they will both improve in muscle strength and hypertrophy.

Muscle fibres used to be classified as either red or white. We can still classify them in that basic way but there is a little bit more to it than that. Although people with a higher percentage of white muscle fibres tend to respond better to resistance training than those with the predominantly higher percentage of red fibres, it must be noted that there is another subdivision of white muscle fibre which can be interchangeable depending on the type of training programme applied. When we look at table number 4, Muscle Fibre Types, if we go through each column in turn we can see that Type I, that's the SO or Slow Twitch Oxidative fibres, these are predominantly the red fibres, which have a slow speed of contraction but they are fatigue resistant. These fibres are utilised more in endurance events. They have a low hypertrophic capability. That means they don't tend to grow and get stronger. They have a high aerobic capacity, mainly due to high levels of myoglobin, so the rate of change of oxygen is really useful for aerobic capacity in endurance events. As you can see, the strength of contraction is low.

MUSCLE FIBRE TYPES					
MUSCLE FIBRE TYPE	FAST OR SLOW TWITCH	FATIGUEABILITY	HYPERTROPHY CAPABILITY	AEROBIC CAPACITY	STRENGTH OF CONTRACTION
RED (ST) · TYPE (1) OXIDATIVE (SO)	(Speed of Contraction) SLOW	FATIGUE RESISTANT	LOW	HIGH	LOW
WHITE (FT) · TYPE (2) a FAST OXIDATIVE GLYCOLYTIC (FOG) ▲ Interchangeable ▲ ▼ through training ▼ TYPE (2) b FAST, GLYCOLYTIC (FG)	FAST	FATIGUEABLE	HIGH	MEDIUM	HIGH
	FAST	MOST FATIGUEABLE	HIGHEST	LOW	HIGHEST

The next two types are under the Type II classification. The Type II classification is the white muscle fibres and, although these can be subdivided further, I'm keeping it simple by dividing them into two groups. The first group is the Type II A. This is the Fast Twitch Oxidative Glycolytic or the FOG fibres. As you can see, these are predominantly Fast Twitch, they're fatigable, they have a high hypertrophic capability, they have a medium aerobic capacity so they last longer than the FG fibres but not as long as the SO fibres, and they have a high strength of contraction. If we compare these to the Type II B, these are the Fast Twitch Glycolytic or FG fibres. These fatigue the quickest but they have the highest power and the highest hypertrophic capability, and a low aerobic capacity. It has been shown under experimental conditions that with regard to the white FT fibres these, as a group, fatigue the quickest, producing the highest lactate levels in the muscle. They also use Creatine Phosphate as an energy substrate primarily, especially the FG fibres. The FG fibres tend to fatigue under maximum load after 30 seconds. The FOG fibres fatigue under maximum load after 60 seconds. Any exercise where the muscle is loaded beyond 60 seconds of continuous tension, the red muscle fibres, or the ST fibres, come into play because the white fibres are fatigued.

If we take all this information into consideration with regard to training techniques we can see that the two types of muscle fibre that hypertrophy the most are the FOG and FG fibres. If we are performing a set, to maximise the response of these fibres, we don't want the set to last longer than 60 seconds so we have to undergo maximum load within that 60 seconds. However, as we see, the FG fibres have the strongest contraction and hypertrophy the most, we can see it is even more useful if the set only lasts for 30 seconds. If we consider one repetition of a high intensity resistance exercise lasts approximately four seconds, with an explosive positive and a controlled negative contraction, this equates to seven to eight repetitions maximum. Therefore, each set, with each repetition performed in four seconds, should be no longer than seven repetitions in duration. There is some justification for a 60 second set to train the FOG fibres, but we'll discuss that more at length in Chapter 5. If we incorporate what we've learnt from the energy systems as well, we can see that in between sets, especially as weight gets heavier, and more motor units are recruited, that we need to leave at least two to three minutes' rest in between sets.

Determining Fibre Type

Since the only way to directly determine the fibre type composition in athletes is to perform an invasive muscle biopsy test (in which a needle is stuck into the muscle and a few fibres are plucked out to be examined under the microscope) some studies have tried to indirectly estimate the fibre type composition of an individual by testing for a relationship between the different properties of fibre type and muscle fibre composition. This type of research has yielded promising results with significant relationships being found between the proportion of FG fibres and muscle strength or power.

An indirect method that can be used in the weight room to determine the fibre composition of muscle groups is as follows;
On a particular exercise, such as bench press, once the muscles have been warmed up adequately, building up the weight slowly and resting long enough in between sets, you ask the athlete to attempt a one rep maximum. Once you establish this maximum weight the athlete can lift for one repetition, he then rests for at least five minutes. Then, ask him to perform as many repetitions with 80% of the one rep max (1RM) as he can. If he does fewer than seven repetitions then the muscle group is likely composed of more than 50% FT fibres. If they can perform twelve or more repetitions then the muscle group has probably more than 50% ST fibres. If the athlete can do between seven and twelve repetitions of 80% of the one RM, then the muscle group probably has an equal proportion of fibres.

| DETERMINING FIBRE TYPE | |
| MUSCLE FIBRE TESTING | |
NO. REPS PERFORMED AT 80% 1RM	MUSCLE FIBRE TYPE
< 7	MOSTLY FAST TWITCH FIBRE DOMINANT (WHITE)
7-10	MIXED FIBRE TYPE
> 10	MOSTLY SLOW TWITCH FIBRE DOMINANT (RED)

Implications For Training

An athlete with a greater proportion of Fast Twitch (FT) fibres will not be able to complete as many repetitions at a given relative amount of weight as will an athlete with a greater proportion of Slow Twitch fibres and, therefore, will never attain as high a level of muscular endurance as will the ST fibred athlete. Similarly, an athlete with a greater proportion of ST fibres will not be able to lift as heavy a weight or run intervals as fast as will an athlete with a greater proportion of FT fibres and, therefore, will never be as strong or as powerful as will the FT fibred athlete. This doesn't mean it's the end of the road as regards strength training for the athlete with more than 50% ST fibres. As this experiment is only a rough determination of fibre type, very often athletes may have a relatively high percentage of FOG fibres which we can still classify as part of the white fibre group. These fibres are interchangeable, i.e. if the training done is predominantly strength and power related training and not endurance training, these fibres will err more on the side of FG fibres, having more Glycolytic capability than Oxidative. These can be trained to hypertrophy similar to FG fibres if given the right training techniques.

Training an FT fibred muscle for endurance will not increase the number of ST fibres, nor will training an ST fibred muscle for strength and power increase the number of FT fibres. For example, an athlete may have a 50/50 mix of FT/ST fibres in a muscle, but since FT fibres normally have a larger cross sectional area than ST fibres, 65 percent of that muscle's area

28

may be FT and 35 percent may be ST. Following a strength training programme for improvement in muscular strength, the number of FT and ST fibres will remain the same (still 50/50) however, the cross sectional area will change. This happens because the ST fibres will atrophy while the FT fibres will hypertrophy (get larger).

Depending on the specific intensity used in training, the muscle may change to a 75 percent FT area and a 25 percent ST area. The change in area will lead to greater strength but decreased endurance capabilities. Since the mass of the FT fibres is greater than that of the ST fibres, the athlete will gain mass and will increase his circumference of the muscle. Conversely, if the athlete trains for muscular endurance, the FT fibres will atrophy while the ST fibres hypertrophy causing a greater area of ST fibres. The area of the muscle which began at 65 percent FT and 35 percent ST before training, may change to 50 percent FT and 50 percent ST following training. The endurance capabilities of the muscle will increase while its strength will decrease and the athlete will lose some muscle mass because ST fibres are lower in mass than FT fibres. The decrease in mass will be observed by a smaller circumference of the muscle.

Chapter 2 - Energy Systems and Muscle Fibre Types Summary

1) Energy from food can produce work, thermal energy or get stored as fat.
2) All activities require energy and ultimately become thermal energy.
3) Athletes with more muscle mass tend to have higher metabolic rates and, therefore, require more energy, i.e. food.
4) The breakdown of larger molecules to smaller ones releasing energy is called CATABOLISM.
5) The synthesis of larger molecules from smaller molecules requires energy and is called ANABOLISM.
6) ATP hydrolyses to produce energy to contract a muscle or to synthesise amino acids into new proteins in muscle cells.

7) Creatine Phosphate (the phosphagen system) produces the initial energy for lifting heavy weights (it lasts for ten seconds).

8) GLYCOLYSIS producing lactate is the second energy system. GLYCOLYSIS requiring oxygen but not producing lactate is the third energy system.

9) Any less intense sustained exercise for longer than ten minutes mainly uses fats (fatty acids) for energy, this is the fourth energy system.

10) Enough time needs to be allowed for the hydrogen ions, lactate and Phosphates to be removed from a muscle before a maximum intensity set is performed. This usually takes three minutes after the last heavy warm up or set.

11) The white muscle fibres (FG and FOG) are the main fibres bodybuilders need to be concerned about with regard to training.

12) FG fibres fatigue after 30 seconds of constant tension, FOG fibres fatigue after about a minute of constant tension. Both these sets of fibres are grouped in the white (FT) class of fibres.

13) FOG fibres can develop more Oxidative (like red fibres) or more Glycolytic (like white fibres) characteristics depending on how they are trained.

14) White fibres (FT) have a larger diameter than red fibres (ST) and have a much stronger contractile force but have much less endurance.

Chapter 3
How A Muscle Repairs and Grows

Introduction

Few fitness professionals and personal trainers are fully aware of the physiological complexity of the factors involved in creating new muscle growth (hypertrophy). Few fitness professionals are well informed as to how muscles adapt and grow to the progressively increasing overload demands of resistance training. In fact, skeletal muscle is the most adaptable tissue in the human body, and muscle hypertrophy (increase in size) is a vastly researched topic and yet is still considered a fertile area of research. This chapter will provide a brief update on some of the more intriguing cellular changes that occur leading to muscle growth. This is referred to as the satellite cell theory of muscle hypertrophy.

Trauma to the Muscle

When muscles undergo intense exercise as from a heavy resistance training regime, there is trauma to the muscle fibres referred to as muscle injury or damage in scientific investigations. This disruption to the muscle cell activates satellite cells which are located on the outside of the muscle fibres. These satellite cells proliferate to the injury site, in essence, as a biological effort to repair or replace damaged muscle fibres. This begins with the satellite cells fusing together with the muscle fibres, often leading to increases in muscle fibre cross sectional area or hypertrophy. These satellite cells have only one nucleus and can replicate by dividing. As the satellite cells multiply, some remain on the muscle fibre, whereas the majority differentiate (the process cells undergo as they mature into normal cells) and fuse to muscle fibres to form new muscle protein strands (myofibrils) and/or repair damaged fibres. Thus, the muscle cells, myofibrils, will increase in thickness and number. The resultant increase in the number of myofibrils tends to lead to a suggestion of an increase in number of muscle fibres via longitudinal fibre splitting as a response to high intensity resistance training. This is known as HYPERPLASIA. Hyperplasia has been shown to occur in animals, but the findings are controversial in human studies.

While hyperplasia cannot be ruled out completely, it does not appear to be the major strategy for muscle tissue adaptation to resistance training. If it occurs at all, it involves only a small amount of the stimulated tissue, maybe less than 10 percent if the conditions are optimal. Thus, the muscle cell's myofibrils will increase in thickness and number. After fusion with the muscle fibre, some satellite cells serve as a source of new nuclei to supplement the growing muscle fibre. With these additional nuclei the muscle fibre can synthesise more proteins and create more contractile myofilaments such as Actin and Myosin in skeletal muscle cells (see Chapter 1). It is interesting to note that high numbers of satellite cells are found associated within Slow Twitch muscle fibres as compared to Fast Twitch muscle fibres within the same muscle as the slow switch fibres are regularly going through cell maintenance repair from daily activities, whereas the Fast Twitch muscle fibres tend to need to be repaired more with heavy duty resistance training.

Growth Factors

Growth factors or hormones are hormone-like compounds called peptide compounds that stimulate satellite cells to produce the gains in the muscle fibre size. These growth factors have been shown to affect muscle growth by regulating satellite cell activity. Hepatocyte growth factor (HGF) is a key regulator in satellite cell activity. It has been shown to be the active factor in damaged muscle and may also be responsible for causing satellite cells to migrate to the damaged muscle area. Fibroblast growth factor (FGF) is another important growth factor in muscle repair following exercise.

The role of FGF may be in the revascularisation (forming new blood capillaries) process during muscle regeneration. A great deal of research has been focused on the role of growth hormone (GH) and IGF-1 (Insulin-like growth factor 1) and it's isoforms in muscle growth. Growth hormone (GH) is made in the anterior pituitary gland in the brain. It is then released into the bloodstream where it stimulates the liver to produce IGF-1 (Insulin-like growth factor 1). IGF-1 levels are increased by protein intake and glucose, and also by high resistance exercise. Production is also regulated by insulin. IGF-1 has a growth promoting effect on almost every cell of the body but especially in muscle, cartilage, bone and nerve cells.

As the name insulin-like growth factor implies, IGF-1 is structurally related to insulin and can also bind to insulin receptors in cells. IGF-1 plays a primary role in regulating the amount of muscle mass growth, promoting changes occurring in the DNA for protein synthesis, and promoting muscle cell repair. Insulin also stimulates muscle growth by enhancing protein synthesis and facilitating the entry of glucose into cells. The satellite cells use glucose as a fuel substrate, thus enabling their cell growth activities. Glucose is also used for intramuscular energy needs. Insulin is the peptide hormone produced by the pancreas and has the effect of increasing glucose uptake and storage from the bloodstream. Glucose is stored in the form of glycogen in the liver and the muscles, and is used as a primary energy source for muscle contraction. Insulin also increased the protein synthesis in cells and it inhibits proteolysis (the breakdown of body protein).

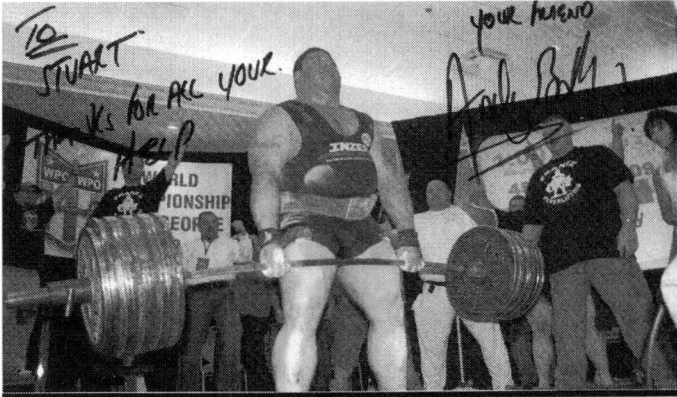

ANDY "THE JACK" BOLTON
First man in history to break the 1000lb barrier
455kg, -1003lb World Record Deadlift

Proud to have been his Physio and adviser through his most prolific period.

In a nutshell, it helps increase muscle hypertrophy (anabolism) and decreases muscle loss (catabolism). Testosterone also affects muscle hypertrophy. This hormone can stimulate growth hormone responses in the pituitary gland which enhances amino acid uptake and protein synthesis in skeletal muscle. In addition, testosterone can increase the presence of neurotransmitters at the fibre site which can help to activate tissue growth. As a steroid hormone, testosterone can interact with nuclear receptors on the DNA resulting in protein synthesis. Testosterone also has a regulatory effect on satellite cells.

MGF (Mechano Growth Factor)

The systemic variant of IGF-1 is produced in the liver. However, recent studies have shown that, locally, within the muscle, at least two other variations or isoforms of IGF-1 are produced. One of these is called MGF, or Mechano Growth Factor. Professor Goldspink, in London, who did some studies during the last decade, has found that a significant amount of MGF was produced directly in the muscle after a single bout of high load eccentric or negative resistance training. Also, in 2006, Dreyer et al. published the result of a study which compared the satellite response of an eccentric exercise regime with a standard concentric programme. It was found that the muscle that underwent the slow, negative contraction produced more muscle damage following exercise and subsequently produced an increase in satellite cell recruitment to the area. This also resulted in a dramatic increase of Mechano Growth Factor (MGF) to the area.

All these factors resulted in a massive increase in muscle protein synthesis and the repair and subsequent hypertrophy of the muscle concerned. It was also noted in different studies that eccentric training also produced an increased turnover of collagen in collagen fibres in tendons. This resulted in increased tensile stress and an improvement in repair due to overuse. More research needs to be done to see the correlation between increased expressions of MGF and whether or not this plays a role in the collagen synthesis also.

35

Myostatin

Myostatin is also known as growth differentiation factor 8, (GDF-8). It is a protein produced and released by myocytes that act on muscle cells to inhibit myogenesis, which is the muscle cell growth and differentiation. It is encoded by the MSTN gene. Animals that either lack Myostatin or are treated with substances that block the activity of Myostatin have significantly more muscle mass. Furthermore, individuals who have mutations in both copies of the Myostatin gene have significantly more muscle mass and are stronger than normal. There is hope that studies into Myostatin may have therapeutic application in treating muscle wasting diseases such as muscular dystrophy. Myostatin was discovered in 1997 by geneticists Se-Jin Lee and Alexandra McPherron who produced a strain of mice that lacked the gene, and had approximately twice as much muscle as normal mice. These mice were subsequently named mighty mice. Naturally occurring deficiencies of Myostatin of various sorts have been identified in some humans.

Double Muscled Cattle

After that discovery, several laboratories cloned and established the nucleotide sequence of a Myostatin gene in two breeds of cattle, the Belgian Blue and the Piedmontese. Unlike the mice with the damaged Myostatin gene, these cattle breeds exhibited muscle cells that multiply rather than enlarge. People describe these cattle breeds as double muscled, but the total increase in all the muscles is no more than 40 percent. Animals lacking Myostatin, or animals treated with substances such as follistatin, that block the binding of Myostatin to its receptor, have significantly larger muscles. Thus, reduction of Myostatin could potentially benefit the livestock industry with even a 20 percent reduction in Myostatin levels, potentially having a large effect on the development of muscles.

Belgian Blue Bull

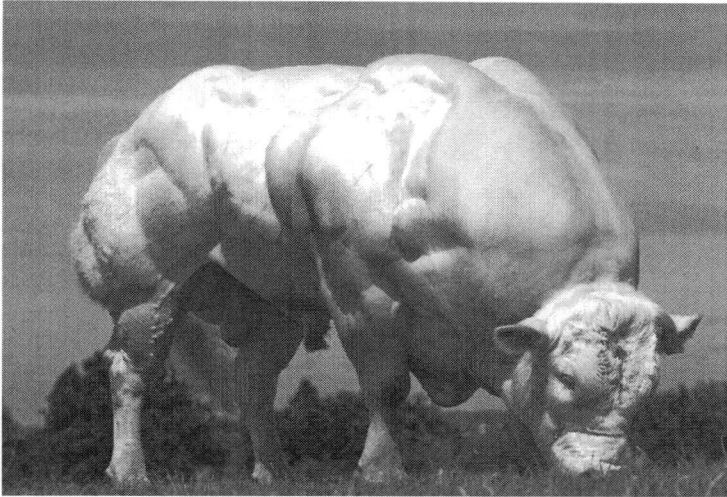

In Humans

A technique for detecting mutations in Myostatin variants has been developed. Mutations that reduce the production of Myostatin lead to an overgrowth of muscle tissue. Myostatin related muscle hypertrophy has an incomplete autosomal dominance pattern of inheritance. People with mutation in both copies of the gene (homozygotes) have significantly increased muscle mass and strength. People with a mutation in one copy of the gene in each cell (heterozygotes) have increased muscle bulk but to a lesser degree. It was discovered in 2004 and 2005 in a German boy and an American boy, and it is likely that in some top level bodybuilders they either have a mutation in one copy or both copies of the genes. This would lead to a predisposition to putting on at least 40 percent muscle than the average human male. As of 2012 no Myostatin inhibiting drugs for humans are on the market. Some of these drugs are currently under development but will take many years to develop to a stage where they could be used for conditions such as muscular dystrophy. Some athletes, eager to get their hands on such drugs, turn to the internet where fake Myostatin blockers are being sold. Temporary reductions of Myostatin levels can be produced by certain easily available products, one of these is Creatine supplementation. Some studies have also shown that IGF-1 and Mechano Growth Factor (MGF) may also concurrently increase protein synthesis partly due to suppression of Myostatin.

The ACE Gene

Although it is widely accepted that genetics play a large role in sports performance, the exact genotypes that can predict elite athletic ability are still very unclear. Perhaps the most well studied gene in respect of sports performance is the Angiotensin Converting Enzyme (ACE) which converts angiotensin I to angiotensin II in muscle. Low levels of ACE activity are observed in athletes that have a predisposition for endurance performance through changes in blood pressure and cardiovascular function. High levels of ACE activity are observed in athletes that have a predisposition to strength and power ability. ACE causes an Actin binding protein to be enhanced in type II (white muscle fibres). Loss of this protein is thought to make type II fibres weaker or slower. Therefore, people with higher ACE levels are thought to display superior strength and power ability for this reason.

Muscle Fibre Changes

Muscle Fibres, especially the white Type II high threshold motor units, must be activated in order to stimulate hypertrophy. During resistance training, both Type I (red) and Type II (white) muscle fibres are recruited and are, therefore, presented with a potent stimulus for adaptation. Resistance training typically increases both Type I (red) and Type II (white) muscle fibre area. This fibre hypertrophy translates into increases in the CSA (Cross Sectional Area) of the intact muscle after several months of training. However, muscle fibre hypertrophy does not occur uniformly between the two major fibre types. It has been shown that Type II fibres manifest greater increases in size than

Type I fibres. In fact, it has been argued that the ultimate potential for hypertrophy may reside in the relative proportion of Type II (white fibres) within a given athlete's muscles. That is, athletes who genetically possess a relatively larger proportion of Fast Twitch (white) fibres may have a greater potential for increasing muscle mass with resistance training than individuals possessing predominantly Slow Twitch (red) fibres.

The pattern of neural stimulation to a muscle dictates that the muscle fibres contract from the most Oxidative to the least Oxidative type. This means that the Type I red fibres contract first and the highest threshold white fibres (the FG fibres) contract last. This is based on the size principle that we'll speak about in the chapter on neural adaptations. Although the proportions of Type I (red) and Type II (white) fibres are genetically determined, changes within each subtype can occur with anaerobic or aerobic training. The changes in the Fast Twitch fibre types can occur between the FOG Type II fibres and the FG Type II fibres. It has been found that overstimulation of the FG fibres can lead to a change back into an FOG fibre type. An example of this would be an athlete performing multiple maximum load sets, probably with less rest in between each set, stimulating the Oxidative capacity of the muscle fibre and causing the Type II white fibres that are classed as FG to change into FOG to accommodate the demand. Although both FOG and FG fibres are attributed to hypertrophy of the muscle, it is the higher threshold less Oxidative FG fibres that are responsible more for power, strength and hypertrophy.

It's interesting to note that in some studies done, during a period of detraining, when the athlete was resting, the proportion of FG fibres actually increased. This is useful to know when determining if an athlete is over-trained or not. If muscle hypertrophy and power and strength decrease on a particular regime, it might be useful to reassess rest periods in between workouts. Although white fibres can change from FOG to FG and vice versa, it is unlikely that Type I red fibres can change to Type II white fibres. Having said this, further studies need to be done. It will be interesting to see if a marathon runner followed

39

a high intensity resistance training programme or a power lifter begins an extensive aerobic endurance programme to see if there was any shift from Type I to Type II and vice versa.

Another adaptation with heavy resistance training is the reduction of mitochondrial density in the trained muscles. Mitochondria in the cells are responsible for respiration and energy exchange. Although the number of mitochondria may remain constant or increase, the mitochondrial density is expressed relative to muscle area. Consequently, the density of mitochondria decreases with muscle hypertrophy. Muscle hypertrophy also results in decreased capillary density by similar mechanisms, although the number of capillaries per fibre may increase. This affects blood flow and Oxidative capacity of the muscle overall when compared to Type I (red) muscle fibres. Most of the mitochondrial and capillary density reduction occurs in the FG fibres. As a result of this, lactate levels can rise in muscles when performing heavy resistance exercise. It is, therefore, useful to try and encourage stimulation of the FOG fibres within the white fibre range by improving the buffering capacity or the removal of lactate from the muscle and the stimulation of capillary density by doing high intensity interval training. This could be done using a TABATA style process which involves high intensity short duration bursts followed by short rests to improve the anaerobic threshold of the muscle. As long as this is done in short duration events with rest periods in between, maybe two to three times a week maximum, there should be no interruption in the overall improvement of the size of the muscle.

Connective Tissue Adaptations

The term connective tissue incorporates tendons, ligaments, fascia and cartilage. These are all complex and dynamic structures that are the critical link between muscles and bones. The primary structural component of all these connective tissues is collagen. The primary stimulus for the growth and increase in strength of tendons, ligaments and fascia is the mechanical forces created during resistance exercise. The degree of tissue

40

adaptation appears to be proportional to the intensity of the exercise. Consistent resistance exercise that exceeds the threshold of strain stimulates connective tissue changes. Evidence suggests that connective tissues must increase their functional capabilities in response to increased muscle strength and hypertrophy. The sites where connective tissues can increase strength and load bearing capacity are;

1) At the junction between the tendon (and ligament) and the bone surface;
2) Within the body of the tendon or ligament and;
3) In the network of fascia within skeletal muscle.

Stronger muscles pull with greater force on their bony attachments and cause an increase in bone mass at the tendon bone junction and along the line over which the forces are distributed. The adaptation that occurs at the tendon bone junction is quite effective. High intensity resistance training results in connective tissue growth and other ultrastructural changes that enhance force transmission. Specific changes within a tendon that contribute to its increase in size and strength include;

1) An increase in collagen fibril diameter;
2) A greater number of cross links within the hypertrophied fibre;
3) An increase in the number of collagen fibrils and;
4) An increase in the packing density of the collagen fibrils.

Collectively, these adaptations increase the tendon's ability to withstand greater tensional forces. Muscle hypertrophy also relates to an increase in the number and size of fibroblasts. Fibroblasts are the main cells in connective tissue, whose main function is to release matrix proteins like collagens which then maintain the structural integrity of the tissue they supply. Increasing the number and size of these fibroblasts results in a greater supply of total collagen. This may explain why biopsies of trained athletes have shown that hypertrophied muscle contains greater total collagen. Recent studies indicate that

41

tendon stiffness increases as a result of this and as a result of resistance training.

One thing that must be emphasised though is the difference in vascularisation of muscles compared to tendons and ligaments. Muscles in general, even Type II fibres, have a relatively high blood flow and rate of turnover when compared to tendons and ligaments. They, therefore, repair much quicker than ligaments and tendons. This needs to be considered when undergoing Glycolytic intense training regimes. If persistently exposed to high levels of resistance, without chance for recovery, degradation of the tendon and ligament structures may ensue. This can lead to injury. In order to prevent this, adjustments to the training regime need to be made. Introduction of slow negative (eccentric) training is a good way to stimulate the growth factors and the fibroblasts required to maintain the integrity of the tendons and ligaments. We will discuss this in a later chapter on periodisation and training protocols.

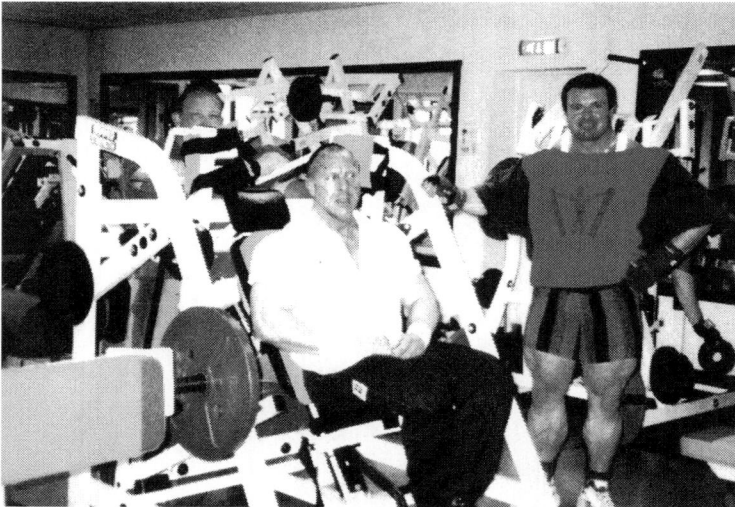

The' Gruesome Threesome!!': Brian, Pat and Myself training in my Gym in Atherton, Manchester.

1) Satellite Cell Theory

HOW A MUSCLE REPAIRS AND GROWS

INTENSE RESISTANCE EXERCISE

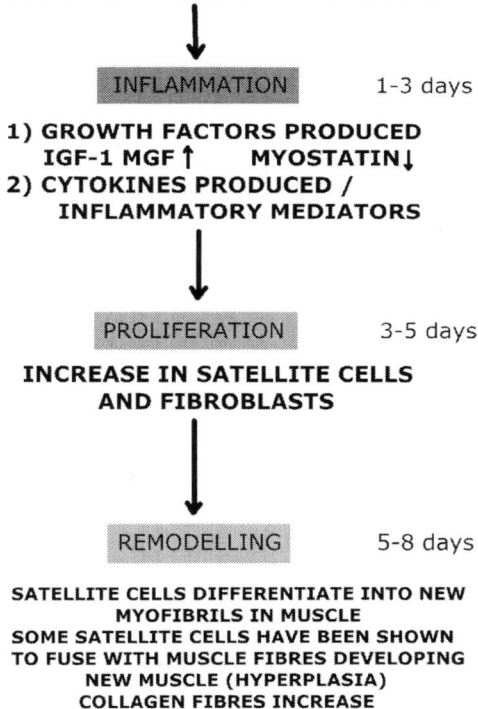

↓

| INFLAMMATION | 1-3 days |

1) GROWTH FACTORS PRODUCED
IGF-1 MGF ↑   MYOSTATIN↓
2) CYTOKINES PRODUCED /
INFLAMMATORY MEDIATORS

↓

| PROLIFERATION | 3-5 days |

INCREASE IN SATELLITE CELLS
AND FIBROBLASTS

↓

| REMODELLING | 5-8 days |

SATELLITE CELLS DIFFERENTIATE INTO NEW
MYOFIBRILS IN MUSCLE
SOME SATELLITE CELLS HAVE BEEN SHOWN
TO FUSE WITH MUSCLE FIBRES DEVELOPING
NEW MUSCLE (HYPERPLASIA)
COLLAGEN FIBRES INCREASE

As you can see from the table above, no training should be attempted on the same body part following a workout for five days, even when the delayed onset muscle soreness has gone you are still just entering the remodelling phase and enough time needs to have elapsed for the satellite cells to differentiate into new muscle. Arthur Jones, in his early books, did some studies with a MedX machine which proved that even after 14 days there was no loss of muscle tissue from the body part trained.

2) The ACE Gene. High levels of ACE lead to an increase in a protein that strengthens Type II white fibres.

3) Both Type I and Type II fibres increase in size with intense resistance training, but Type II proportionally increase more.

4) Muscle fibres contract, Type I fibres first and then through to Type II (ST → FOG → FG).

5) FOG fibres can change to FG fibres and vice versa, dependent on the type of training done.

6) As white muscle fibres get bigger, their strength/power increases but their aerobic capacity decreases.

7) Short bursts of high intensity TABATA style training can help the speed of removal of lactate from the muscle and improve circulatory supply.

8) Connective tissues such as tendons and ligaments also increase in strength when subjected to high intensity resistance training.

9) Tendons (and ligaments) need longer to recover after heavy resistance exercise than muscles to prevent injury. This needs to be factored into training regimes i.e. periods of rest, eccentric exercise, higher reps or a combination of all three.

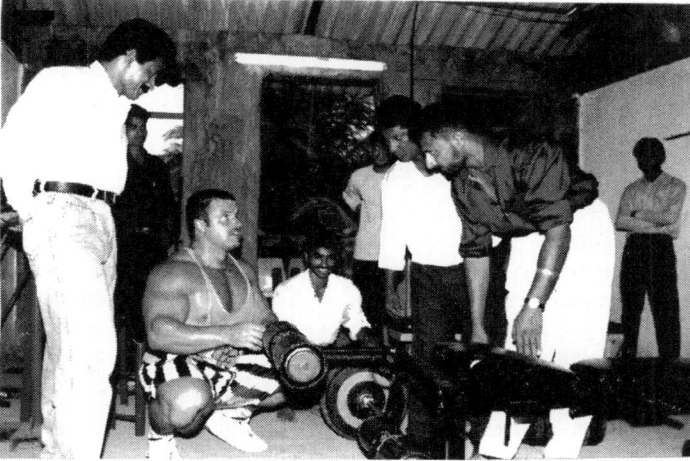

Myself coaching bodybuilders in Goa, India during the 90's. I did a series of seminars over there over a 4 year period.

Chapter 4
Neural Adaptation to Weight Training

All movements start in your brain. An area in the brain, called the motor cortex, produces signals that travel down your spinal cord. This travels off down peripheral nerves which then eventually form into motor neurons to supply muscle fibres. As we have already learnt, the motor unit, i.e. the motor neuron supplying its respective muscle fibres is the main system we wish to activate to produce muscle contraction. The smallest motor units, i.e. the nerve fibres supplying the least number of muscle fibres are primarily the Slow Twitch Oxidative fibres, or the red fibres. These fibres are more involved in endurance activities. These fibres require the lowest threshold of force for activation. They also have the lowest rate of impulse firing. In contrast, the largest motor units are the FG Fast Twitch Glycolytic muscle fibres. These are the largest of the white muscle fibres and have the highest threshold of force in order to activate them. They also have the fastest firing of impulses per second.

The FOG fibres, or Fast Twitch Oxidative Glycolytic, are the fibres that lie in the middle. They still respond to heavy training and have a relatively high threshold and firing rate. As you have probably figured out so far, it's of benefit to anybody involved in bodybuilding and strength training that we fire up as many of the large motor units as possible within a given time under tension. There is a particular principle called the Henneman Size Principle, this states that motor units are recruited in an orderly manner from the smallest to the largest, and that recruitment is dependent on the effort and the force of the activity. It stands to reason that a heavier weight when applied to a particular muscle will recruit more motor units, but if you have the muscle contracting isometrically, i.e. statically, against an immovable force, then the amount of motor unit recruitment is dependent on the effort sustained. More effort involves more motor unit recruitment and the force applied then will be

46

greater. Although the Henneman principle can be applied across the board to weight training and most power sports, occasionally it is observed that there are a few exceptions to this Size Principle. It has been observed that during very rapid changes of direction in force production and ballistic muscular contractions, such as plyometric box jumping or a sudden change of direction in sports such as rugby, that selective recruitment of Fast Twitch motor units may occur with an inhibition in lower threshold motor units. If we increase the force from low to high, the motor unit recruitment involves larger motor units, but we also see that if the force contraction is faster, then more motor units are recruited. Looking at diagram 4, not only are more motor units recruited when the force goes from low to high, but also the firing rate of those motor units increases. As you can see with the FG fibres, when the percentage of maximum contraction goes from 60 to nearly 100 percent, the rate of firing dramatically increases to 70 impulses per second.

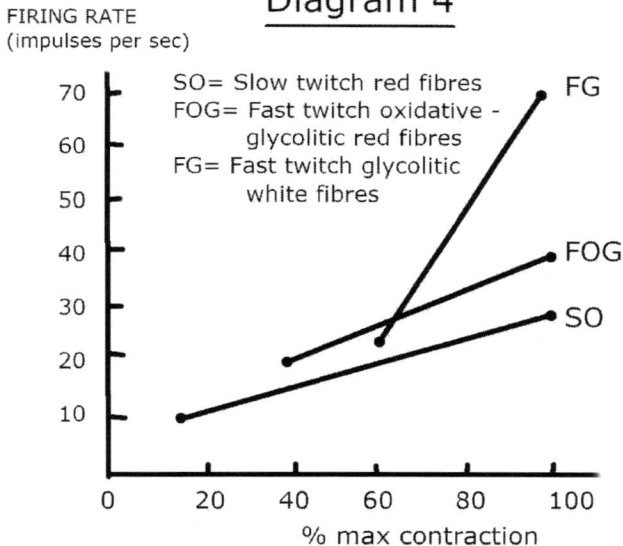

There are two basic ways to lift. Lift as heavy as possible and lift as fast as possible. Now, keep in mind that heavy weights won't move quickly no matter how hard you try, but they don't need to. When the weight is heavy enough to allow only a few repetitions you're recruiting all your motor units because it takes every ounce of effort to get the weight moving. As long as when you attempt to lift the weight you attempt to lift it as fast as possible concentrically, or in the shortening phase of the movement, then you will recruit your maximum number of motor units.

Where many trainers make a mistake is with submaximal weights. Here we're talking about lighter weights that you could move faster but don't. If you use a lighter weight, with a slow concentric contraction, you're probably only recruiting about 60 percent of your maximum number of motor units. If you pause at the bottom of the movement and then attempt to accelerate the lift from the first rep as fast as possible, you tap into more motor units that are available. It has also been noted in studies that following an explosive concentric contraction a slow eccentric contraction, or a slow lowering of the weight, maintains more motor unit recruitment once it's been initiated with the initial explosive effort.

Another reason for not performing a concentric contraction slowly is that ischemia may result. This is because a slow positive concentric contraction following a slow negative eccentric contraction will start to cause a shutdown in blood supply to the muscle. This means a lack of oxygen, it also means an increase in lactate levels. Also, the build-up of phosphate from the breakdown of Creatine Phosphate reduces cross bridge formation and calcium reuptake which reduces the contractibility of the muscle. Hydrolysis of ATP also causes Hydrogen Ion increase, which increases the acidity of the muscle, which also inhibits the nerve muscle connection to function properly. This is another reason to rest adequately in between sets to allow the lactic acid to be reabsorbed and reconverted back into energy again, and also the repletion of ATP and Creatine Phosphate also takes longer than one minute.

If a set is performed too quickly without adequate rest then maximum motor unit recruitment is impossible and, therefore, maximum time under tension is impossible for stimulating the muscle to grow. People these days tend to rush through their routines, clock-watching whilst training. It's also a common misconception that if you're taking longer than an hour to do your weight training programme then you're overtraining. People that train this way are forgetting the main concept of weight training, that it's not an endurance event, you're trying to hypertrophy muscle and increase it in strength and fatiguing it aerobically is not the way forward.

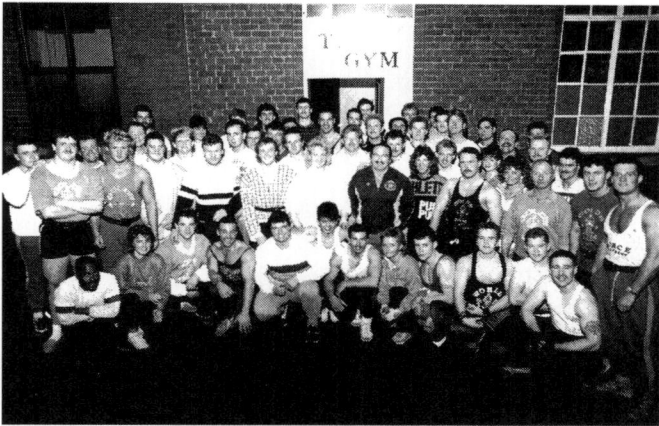

Tim O' Brien simply ran the best gym in Bolton for 20 years during the 80's and 90's. Here we all are in 1987, a 'motley crew!!'

We've already mentioned that in order to recruit as many motor units as possible we need to increase the weight or the load on the bar or on the muscle. However, the decision to apply effort and generate enough force to overcome that weight is totally down to the mental effort or the application of that effort to produce the lift. When a person first starts weight training his neuromuscular system is not geared up to maximise the effort needed. A lot of the muscle activity would be used to help to maintain balance, balance both of his core and the weight being lifted. This requires a lot more effort in the novice weightlifter. A lot of the effort and force required to do this takes up a lot of energy that should be transferred into initiating the prime movers, or the main muscles concerned, to lift the weight. It takes a number of weeks, sometimes months, for this neural adaptation to be good enough to lift the weight more efficiently. It's often noted in novice weightlifters that the ability to lift the weight improves dramatically during this time without any changes in muscle structure. This is because as the neuromuscular system becomes more efficient the novice weightlifter can lift the weight easier without undergoing morphological changes to the muscle, these come later on. What takes even longer, sometimes years, is for the bodybuilder to focus his effort so that he can concentrate on the main prime movers he wants to train to maximise his motor unit recruitment. Not only does he want to maximise the number of motor units, but also he wants to increase the firing rate of the motor units that respond most to the weights. These are the Fast Twitch Glycolytic fibres.

It takes a lot of concentration to try to improve the firing rate of these Fast Twitch Glycolytic fibres. There is a way to measure this. Interpolated Twitch Technique (ITT) is a way to measure muscle activation by applying an electrical current to a muscle already undergoing a maximum voluntary contraction. If any additional force is detected on applying this electrical stimulus, then it is concluded that the Maximum Voluntary Contraction (MVC) was not a true maximum contraction. In other words, the muscle still had some strength left in it that the owner could not voluntarily illicit. It's generally agreed in the scientific community that most athletes cannot contract all their motor units 100 percent. You've probably heard of the stories of eight stone females lifting cars off their trapped spouses. This adrenaline fight/flight response obviously maximises more motor unit recruitment than could be otherwise done voluntarily. If we can somehow tap into this reserve then this would obviously benefit muscle strength and hypertrophy. One of the methods that we use in training, which can tap into this reserve to a degree, is when we perform the primer set before the main working set.

As mentioned earlier, it's very important to have a good blood supply to oxygenate the tissues involved in muscle contraction, i.e. the nerve fibres and the muscle fibres. Warming up prior to the working set is a gradual process of improving capillary network flow, so we improve the blood supply, and then also to slowly increase the recruitment of these motor units prior to what we might consider to be the main event, the working set. One of the things we realise now from the motor cortex, the area in the brain that activates this nervous system, is that once we achieve a maximum, or a near to maximum contraction, the motor cortex remembers this level of motor unit activation. Once it memorises this the motor units are recruited much more quickly and the overall net effort produces a stronger muscle contraction when we come to do the working set. So the idea with the primer set is to be as close as possible to the maximum working set weight without over-fatiguing oneself. Once warmed up, the primer set should involve no more than two or three repetitions with close to the maximum weight you will use for your set, and then adequately resting to allow the muscle to recover its strength, ready for its all-out effort. A typical time period of rest after the primer set, before you do the working set, is two to three minutes. This allows for the lactate and the phosphate to be reconverted and reabsorbed, and the muscle will be in a much better state to undergo maximum contraction.

The Stress Response

One of the things we need to realise is that the neuromuscular system is a very fine tuned system. When it's functioning well it is very efficient, but because there are so many dependant factors to provide this efficient response, if any one of these factors is affected, the whole system can break down. As the system is governed by the brain and the brain is dependent upon hormonal and chemical responses, this can then affect the peripheral nervous system strongly. In other words, if a person is subject to a lot of stress, be that mental, emotional or physical stress, the resultant hormonal response can affect the nerve supply to the peripheral system. As we see from the diagram, stress in its many forms can affect or fatigue the nerve cells. Fatigue of these vasomotor nerve cells causes a relaxation of blood vessel walls, which slows down the rate of blood flow. This can cause postural changes in the fascial tissues of the muscles, it can cause the muscles to weaken, and then this can also result in biomechanical dysfunction. Biomechanical dysfunction causes postural changes which can then increase anoxic pain because of alteration of blood flow. This can then become a vicious circle causing more stress which causes more anoxic pain, which causes more loss of function. I think the main conclusion to come to with regard to the stress response is that it's so important to get adequate rest, nutrition and to deal with any postural changes which may affect the neuromuscular system. We will deal with a lot of these in the chapter entitled, "What prevents a Muscle Responding," and also the chapter covering, "Common Conditions Affecting Bodybuilders," chapters eight and nine.

Chapter Four – Neural Adaption to Weight Training – Summary

1. As force/effort are applied to a muscle, motor units are recruited from small to large, i.e. from slow Oxidative (red fibres) to Fast Twitch Glycolytic FG white fibres. This is called the Henneman Principle.
2. There are occasional exceptions to the Henneman rule. These are where plyometric or sudden changes in direction of force are applied to a muscle, resulting in instant recruitment of large motor units over small motor units.
3. Large motor units are more readily activated when the muscle is attempted to be contracted very quickly. So the goal in training is fast concentric with heavy weights combined with slow eccentric training.
4. Adequate rest needs to be taken in between sets in order to reduce the acidity/lactate levels in the muscle which can cause a shutdown in circulation

and an inhibition of the nerve muscle connection. It also allows for reabsorption of phosphate and repletion of ATP and Creatine levels. The rest period also allows the stress response to be downgraded. This results in the better activation of the motor units for the next set.

5. It takes a few weeks for a novice weightlifter to achieve an adequate neuromuscular adaptation to allow him to focus on lifting the weight more directly. It takes even longer, sometimes many years, for a trainer to focus his efforts in order to recruit as many motor units as possible and also increase the firing rate of the white muscle fibres, resulting in more force recruitment.

6. Performing a primer set prior to the main working set results in maximum activation of motor units in the shortest possible time.

7. Overall, maximum motor unit recruitment depends not only on the weight applied to the muscle, but also to the effort applied by the individual. This requires a great deal of focus and what we call the mind muscle connection. This also can take years of training. This kind of low volume maximum intensity training is not for the fainthearted, and is not, repeat, not an easy option.

8. There is no doubt that neural adaptation plays an important role in the overall adaptation to strength training. When a new training exercise is introduced into the programme, neural adaptation will predominate in the first several weeks of training as the athlete masters the coordination necessary to perform the exercise efficiently. Other adaptations, such as the ability to fire motor units at very high rates to achieve maximal rate of force development require a longer period of time in training to attain, and are also lost more rapidly during detraining. The role of the nervous system should not be ignored when desiring to gain maximum muscle development.

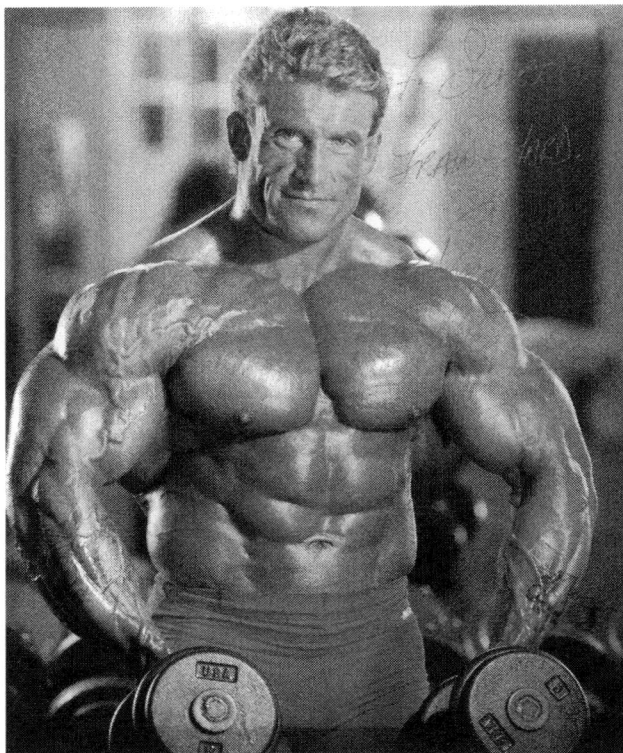

Dorian Yates: 6 Times Mr Olympia winner. Apart from being his Physio for 9 years during his most prolific period, we trained together and discussed training protocols on many occasions. Dorian was one of the few bodybuilders I could talk to in depth on nutrition and muscle physiology. He knew how important it was to make that mind/muscle connection count to achieve his goals. Dorian was the first to help me realise that I used to overtrain. He, along with Arthur Jones, Ellington Darden and Brian Johnston were the biggest influences on the adaptation of these training principles in this book!

Chapter 5
Bodybuilding Methods Through the Ages

When you look back at the history of resistance training, it dates back over 2,000 years from the days of Milo, who was a five-time Olympic games winner in ancient Greece. He employed progressive resistance training and also periodisation, varying the weight and the reps and the regularity of his training to some degree. Over many years, numerous weight training systems have been developed, some merging with others and some even repeating themselves as we go through the decades. It almost appears like it's similar to the fashion industry which tends to go round in circles again and again. This chapter takes us through the history of modern progressive resistance training, dating back from the 1920s, and catalogues the sort of training regimes that were involved. So in this chapter we're just stating the facts about each system and then in the next chapter after this one we'll start to dissect them scientifically and try to analyse the systems to try and attain as near perfect a training regime as is possible. Most of these systems that will be explained now are mainly for bodybuilding purposes although there is some that can be adapted for powerlifting and weightlifting purposes. Obviously, resistance exercises are also useful in relation to sports that involve a degree of strength and power.

1930s Static Contraction Training

What was popularised in the 1930s with Charles Atlas and the dynamic tension training regime came full circle in the 1990s with Peter Sisco's publication of static contraction training. This led to functional isometric movement in training today. Although there were many years between these two systems, isometric based contraction training never really went away, it was just incorporated with isotonic training later on. We start with a brief history of Charles Atlas.

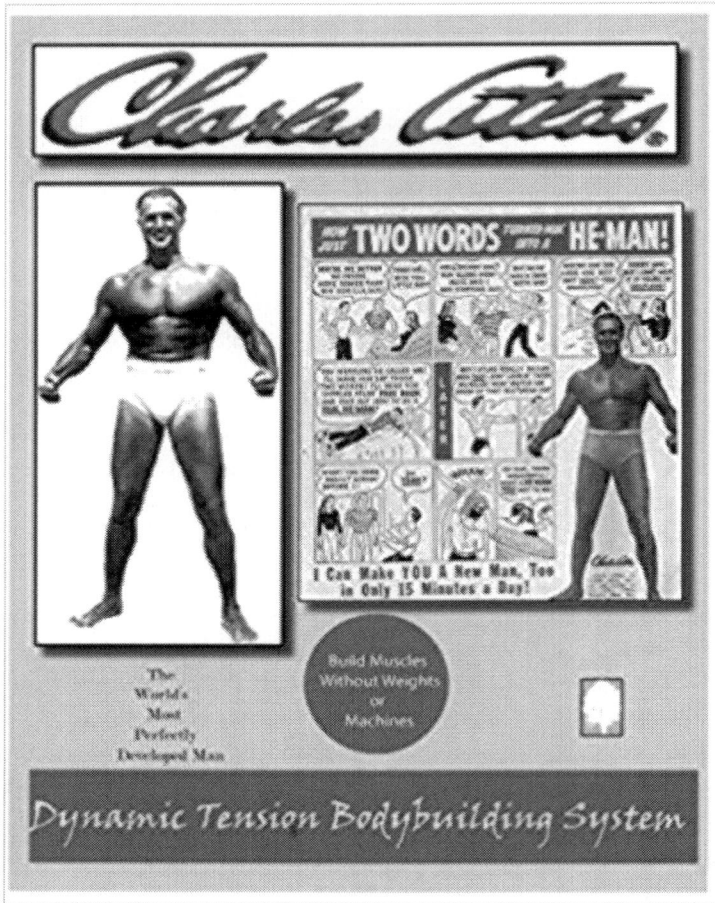

Charles Atlas was an Italian-American bodybuilder, best remembered for developing the bodybuilding method dynamic tension. Atlas trained himself to develop his body from that of a scrawny weakling eventually becoming the most popular bodybuilder of his day. He took the name Charles Atlas after a friend told him that he resembled the statue of Atlas on top of a hotel on Coney Island. He legally changed his name in 1922. He marketed his first bodybuilding course in 1922. Charles

Atlas Limited was founded in 1929. So the story goes, the origin of dynamic tension dated right back to when Atlas was 15 years old. A bully kicked sand into his face on a beach when he was sunbathing and he went back home, looked at himself in the mirror and decided to do something about his life and his physique. He also observed lions at the zoo in New York and he thought to himself, "How does this lion maintain its muscle mass when it doesn't have any barbells or any exercises?" Then it came over him as he began to see the lion stretching continuously and holding muscles tight, pitting one against another. It caused him to think about the role of antagonistic muscle contractions, i.e. contracting one muscle against another, allowing the other one to relax. He decided to develop an exercise regime for all the major muscle groups of the body, incorporating these isometric tension exercises. The dynamic tension program consists of twelve lessons and then one final perpetual lesson. Each lesson was supplemented by photos of Atlas demonstrating the exercises. His products and lessons have sold millions and Atlas became the face of fitness. Among the people who took Atlas' course were; Rocky Marciano, heavyweight boxing champion from 1952 to 1956; Joe Louis, heavyweight boxing champion from 1937 to 1949; British heavyweight weightlifting champion, and Darth Vader actor, David Prowse; and also Alan Wells, the 1980 Moscow Olympic games hundred metre champion. This type of training does not use the traditional system of repetitions. Instead, it only deals with isometric contractions for five to ten seconds using an immovable weight that you use in the strongest range of motion for a particular movement. So usually the midrange. A modern idea to incorporate it into a program would be, for example, in the bench press. If somebody could bench press 220lb for six to eight reps, you might select 280lb for a static contraction weight, holding the loaded bar approximately two to three inches below the lockout position for five to ten seconds. Power lifters have used this type of training for years and they often call it pin pressing. This is where they press the bar against the top pins in a power rack with as much force as possible for six to eight seconds. Martial arts practitioners, including Bruce Lee, have also used this method of training to increase size and strength. Bruce Lee was known to hold a

135lb barbell out in front of his face with straight arms for several seconds.

Static Contraction Training
- Maximum immovable weight
- Very limited or no range of motion
- The effort is based upon time under load and not repetitions

---

The 1950s Volume Training

People like John Grimek and Clarence Ross were the early advocates of volume training back in the 1950s. Volume training can also be abbreviated as HVT or High Volume Training. It consists of numerous sets performed for each muscle group, split routines but frequent training sessions. It's ironic that this is the most common type of weight training observed in gym and fitness centres worldwide today. The volume of work subjected to the body is much greater with this type of training than with other systems that emphasise intensity over volume. The tendency was to employ this system for beginners through to advanced trainers. It was common for the beginners to be given between three to five exercises per muscle group. After one to two years of training they were classed as intermediate and the number of sets was stepped up to maybe six to eight per exercise per body part, and in advanced training, three or more years the number of sets was stepped up to ten to twelve, for the major body parts. Each body part was trained usually two to three times per week. Later on in the late 50s and early 60s a bodybuilder called Vince Gironda, in the states, advocated what became known as the German Volume Training. The goal of German Volume Training is to complete ten sets of ten reps with the same weight on a basic compound movement such as, for example, the bench press, deadlift or squat. Resting intervals were kept to a minimum but were constant. Typically, it would also include two or three assistance exercises, such as, for the chest, incline dumbbell press and the dumbbell fly movement, and these were supplemented on to the

58

compound movement for three sets per exercise. The suggested starting weight for this type of training is 60 percent of your one rep maximum, that's one RM short, in each exercise. For example, if you could squat 300lb for one rep, then your starting weight would be 180lb for ten reps. The same weight would be used on each successive set whilst trying to maintain ten reps per set. As the muscle fatigue accumulates, the temptation to take longer rests rises. However, this system explicitly enforces a constant rest period between sets thus increasing intensity through both the rest interval and increasing loads.

The 1960s PHA – Peripheral Heart Action Training

This training method was developed at the same time that the universal multi-station exercise machines were developed. A guy called Chuck Coker invented these machines and this system was developed as a means by which overall fitness could be achieved with a combination of cardiovascular and resistance training. The main concept of PHA training is to force blood up and down the body by working every major muscle group whilst at the same time maintaining an elevated heart rate. The goal of this training system is to improve strength, muscle size along with cardiovascular efficiency. The main reasoning behind it was to alternately work lower body and upper body exercises so that when the upper body is trained the lower body is resting and vice versa. This can maintain an elevated heart rate whilst giving some degree of rest to muscle groups. The only detriment with this type of training really is that you never really completely rest and the neuromuscular system is always being stressed. However, it's an ideal overall workout if you're short on time and you are just after an overall conditioning of the body. This training concept is by no means limited to universal machines and many fitness emporiums all over the country, both in the UK, Europe and America, adopt this kind of approach as a means by which people can utilise machines in conjunction with a circuit program for overall fitness. Ultimately, maximum hypertrophy and strength cannot be achieved with this system, but it will definitely improve overall muscular endurance.

High Intensity Training (HIT)

The High Intensity Training philosophy was originally developed in the 1960s by Arthur Jones from Nautilus and was later refined and improved by people such as Ellington Darden and Ken Hutchins, amongst others. During the time at which high volume training was very popular, Arthur Jones argued that the opposite is true, that in order to gain muscle size and strength without overtraining, lower volumes, coupled with a High Intensity was the most effective method. He argued that it's impossible to train at High Intensity for a long duration. A classic example would be a sprinter versus a distance runner. A sprinter engages in High Intensity activity, but he cannot maintain that intensity for very long. Conversely, the distance runner is working at a much lower intensity and can, therefore, sustain that level for a much longer duration. Comparing physiques of a marathon runner or a long distance runner with a sprinter it's quite obvious that the person engaging in the High Intensity short duration activity has a much more hypertrophied or developed physique. Many years before Dorian Yates reintroduced the popularity for HIT training, Arthur Jones was advocating the performance of a single High Intensity set to failure for each muscle group. This is, of course, following adequate warm-ups to the area. The most famous experiment ever conducted with regard to this type of training is called the COLORADO EXPERIMENT. This was where a professional bodybuilder, called Casey Viator, gained an incredible 63lb of muscle in only 28 days. Now, this experiment was only ever conducted on two individuals who had previously gained muscle mass from a previous muscle building regime, but had subsequently lost it either due to injury or lay off. So it could be argued that there was a certain degree of muscle memory, especially when we think of Casey Viator who was reasonably genetically gifted as a bodybuilder prior to this experiment, but was regaining quite a lot of this muscle. Having said that, it's an incredible amount of muscle to gain in such a short period of time and can only lend credence to this method of bodybuilding. It must also be added that Arthur Jones and Ellington Darden also insisted that good form be used on exercise. Later on, this High Intensity Training, or HIT training began to be incorporated into the super slow system in the 80s. We'll go on to that later.

Periodisation

Going back to the ancient games, the Greeks used methods of periodisation in their training. In the 1960s, a sports scientist from Russia called Dmitri Matveyev first developed the general training concept of periodisation (cyclic training). He used to map out an entire year's training program through periods of maximal and submaximal work. This method was based on the results of scientific research to discover how best to develop an athlete to their fullest potential. The reasoning behind periodisation was that you cannot train at maximum intensity all the time. This will cause some stagnation in improvement. In order to improve from a plateaued position, an athlete would need to perform different types of work over a period of time. The training program could utilise exercises or regimes to improve muscle power and strength, endurance and functional strength. Matveyev split the whole training year into multiple training cycles;

1) The macrocycle, which encompassed the entire year.
2) Mesocycles which were specific training cycles within the macro cycle. Each one was devoted to a certain, specific purpose such as strength, power or muscular endurance. Typically, these cycles may last six to eight weeks but could be longer or shorter.
3) Microcycle, which is a specific training variation within a mesocycle. Typically, varying the training intensity from day to day.

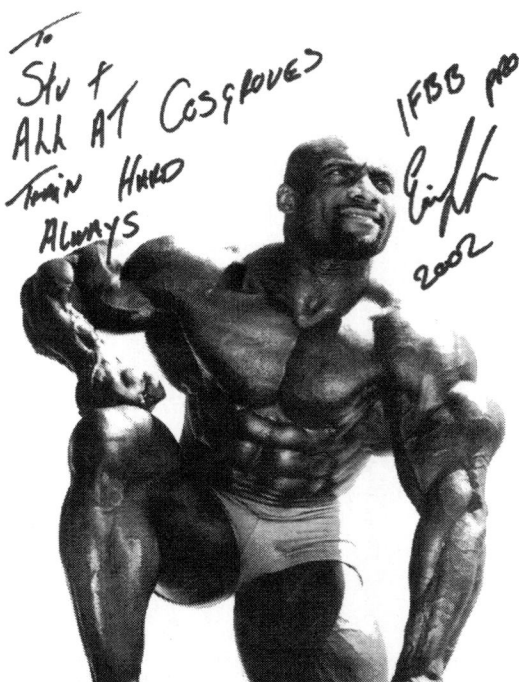

Ernie Taylor: Multiple Title winner, Ernie placed 8th in the 1998 Mr Olympia. Apart from being his Physio,we also had a number of workouts together, especially on legs with Dorian where Ernie utilised these intense low volume sessions to bring his legs up to his amazing upper body!

Bodybuilders in the 70s typically tried to adapt the periodisation principle to train for either strength, muscle hypertrophy or definition, varying the resistance and the repetition range. This seemed to reinforce the concept of different training cycles for muscle mass, muscle shape and definition. Joe Weider reinforced this, mistakenly thinking that certain exercises were responsible more for mass and certain exercises more for definition. During the 70s Arnold is famously depicted in the movie pumping iron after following a phase one of bulking and mass building, undergoing a phase two, which was called cutting and leaning out. The goal here was to maintain the muscle mass built in phase one while reducing your body fat. This phase was typified by the use of moderate weights, super sets and compound giant sets, more volume and more variety of exercises, higher reps and shorter rest periods, with the mistaken belief that you were burning more fat. We now know with modern physiology that weight training doesn't tend to burn fat at a high percentage, it's mainly a glycogen derived energy production. However, it does set up a turnover for long lasting fat metabolism increases for the days ahead. This is more likely to occur training with a more intense program, causing more muscle metabolic turnover, resulting in a longer sustained metabolism for the days ahead.

The Bulgarian Method

During the 70s, members of the Bulgarian national weightlifting team were the dominant weightlifters in the world. It turns out that Bulgarians at the time also were the heaviest anabolic steroid users in the strength world. Ivan Abadjiev, the head coach of the national weightlifting team crafted a training method so sinister that outsiders cringed and insiders called him the butcher. Under his control, the Bulgarian weightlifters trained two to six times per day, six days per week. This is similar to volume orientated bodybuilders of the 60s and 70s who used to train twice a day six days per week. There were no light days, no off season, no periodisation. They trained for specificity. They performed just a few exercises over and over again. Bodybuilders utilise this concept but only for two to four week bursts in order to attempt to attain strength and muscle growth rapidly. Obviously, the main downside to this Bulgarian method was the possibility in overtraining and injuring an athlete more readily than most other systems. It was definitely not for beginners.

Pre-exhaustion Training

Pre-exhaustion training developed in the early 70s. The idea was that you perform a compound movement immediately following a single joint isolation movement. It was initially pioneered by Arthur Jones with his introduction of the HIT training using

Nautilus exercise equipment in the 1960s. For example, in the bench press, the relatively weaker tricep muscles, which assist the press, fail before the pectorals are fully exhausted. With this in mind, a pre-exhaustion exercise such as dumbbell flyes could be done before starting to bench press. This will partially pre-fatigue the chest muscles while keeping the triceps at near full strength. When the bench press is then performed, the tricep muscles are still strong but the chest is then brought to complete fatigue. The key here is to perform the compound exercise immediately after the isolation exercise with little or no rest in between.

Heavy Duty

One of Arthur Jones' early students was a professional bodybuilder called Mike Mentzer who developed the heavy duty training system during the 1970s. Heavy duty was a high intense training philosophy resulting in a maximum effort in a short space of time. Workouts were infrequent, i.e. two per week. The workouts were very short, i.e. 30 minutes. The intensity was as high as possible, with a particular weight involved, i.e. complete eccentric and concentric muscular failure. His main philosophy was the fact that the harder the individual trains the less time he will be able to do it. Therefore intensity and duration exist in an inverse ratio to each other. As Mentzer was listening to Arthur Jones, he recognised that you can train hard or you can train long but you cannot do both. In essence, this is a principle by which Mentzer advocated his famously brief training sessions. Mentzer increased the intensity of the workout by one or more of the following three methods:

1. Progressively increasing the weight used.
2. Progressively decreasing the amount of time required to perform a workout.
3. Performing each set to a point of total muscular failure.

The Weider System

Joe Weider started to develop his system in 1936, but as the years went by and a variety of new weight training methods emerged, Weider selected various principles from each of these, adding these to his metasystem and marketing these concepts using unique names. For instance, what we call negatives, he called the retro-gravity principle. He tried to convert already utilised principles into 'new principles' with his own stamp on them. This was cleverly marketed during the Weider magazine decades from the Muscle Builder in the 50s through to the 70s with Muscle and Fitness and right through to Flex magazine today. You could probably say that the culmination of all these principles first appeared with the publication of the Weider System of Bodybuilding in 1981. It categorised 32 training principles and methods which were developed to try to personalise an individual's goals. However, it must be said that Weider was a staunch believer in advocating volume training and he continued on his merry way as if HIT and heavy duty training never existed. One of the main principles Weider introduced, which nearly everybody utilises these days, is the split principles. This has the athlete dividing the workout week up into separate training sessions targeting specific muscle groups. It could be a two way split, where you work each muscle group twice a week, divided into upper body and lower body. It could be a three way split. This routine has you work each muscle group twice a week but divides the body into three separate workouts based around a push/pull scheme. You're now working out six days a week versus the four days a week in the previous routine. Dividing your workouts into two or three shorter, more intense training sessions per day is Weider's answer to the Bulgarian method, and he called this the double/triple split training principle.

Super Slow

In 1982, an employee of Nautilus was assigned by Arthur Jones to supervise the Nautilus sponsored osteoporosis study at the

University of Florida, College of Medicine. This man was Ken Hutchins and he developed the super slow training system as an exercise system designed to minimise injury whilst maximising intensity. It's designed to make each exercise harder and safer at the same time. Super slow is considered a derivative of the High Intensity Training (HIT) system. Since Arthur Jones concentrated on intensity over form, Hutchins emphasised repetition form as the basis for intensity. Most weight training systems increase the difficulty of the exercise by increasing the weight. This typically increases the acceleration speed in the process using momentum. When you start to handle heavy weights with a lot of momentum this causes the exercise to be potentially more dangerous as you may lose control with the direction of force going outside of your base of support. It's easier to lose control of your car when you're going 100mph versus 10mph. A small shift in the steering wheel at 100mph often produces disastrous results. Similarly, if you were squatting with 400lb+ getting out of your groove could potentially lead to injury and loss of control. Hutchins theorised that if we minimise force during exercise then injury is also often minimised. Since force is determined by mass times acceleration, Hutchins discovered that mass could only be reduced slightly before muscular adaptation failed to occur. In order to maintain enough tension on the muscle, without acceleration, Hutchins advocated that the exercise be done in a slow form format. By slow we mean a six to twelve second interval both on the upward part of the movement and also on the downward part. Any slower and the movement becomes a series of stops and starts, creating a series of accelerations. So in order to maintain constant movement, this six to twelve second interval seemed to be best. The muscle was loaded then constantly in both the concentric and the eccentric portion of the exercise. Obviously, by minimising acceleration and keeping this constant tension, the weight that you're able to lift will be less than normal. Applying super slow to a high volume workout would take absolutely ages. You would be in the gym for hours and would more than likely over-train the whole body in the process. It would be wise to apply super slow within your own workout just on one or two working sets. Physiologically speaking, when we analyse super slow it makes sense on the eccentric part of the movement, but if you perform super slow on both the concentric and the eccentric it can affect blood flow to the muscle. Also, whilst we don't advocate loose accelerative movements in training, it is good to realise that an initial sharp burst of acceleration with a heavy weight causes the stimulation of many more motor units than if the weight is attempted to be lifted slowly. So the initial acceleration on a concentric would maximise motor unit recruitment, and then to try to maintain this motor unit recruitment it makes sense to perform the eccentric part of the movement slowly. So in other words, a hybrid of super slow would tend to work better.

Holistic Training

Dr Fred Hatfield was a famous world champion powerlifter back in the 80s. He set the world record in the squat in the 90kg weight class with a lift of 826lb. He maintained an association with Joe Weider and was a columnist in Muscle and Fitness magazine. This led to his application of periodisation principles into bodybuilding. The result was holistic training. Holistic training centres on the science of muscle cells, where muscles are composed of distinct types of structures. He advocated different types of rep ranges to be applied to four different types of muscle fibre response. He used a variety of rep ranges from three to five, six to ten and 15 plus, for power, size and muscular endurance. He also performed some high rep movements with a slow and continuous tension, attempting to increase the intensity and cause more stress on each of the muscle cell components. He also advocated certain exercises with low reps to be done explosively. He, therefore, combined the different concepts of HIT, periodisation and super slow. One of the bodybuilding champions that practised many of Dr Fred Hatfield's programs was Lee Haney the eight time Mr Olympia champion. Many of these principles that Dr Fred Hatfield advocated have since been proven physiologically. Certainly, when we look at muscle fibre types, there does appear to be different subtypes of white Type II fibres and they do fatigue at different rates. It would make sense that certainly to expose them to differing times under tension, i.e. different rep ranges, would make sense.

Angular Training

Early in the 1990s, a guy called Steve Hallman, who was the former editor of Iron Man magazine, developed a concept of weight training which involved three angular positions which he called the POSITIONS OF FLEXION. This worked each muscle group from three angular positions within the same workout. The three angular positions were the midrange, the stretch and the contraction. If we look at the midrange, if we consider the bicep curl, the midrange is the middle part of the movement around about 90 degrees, where the muscle is neither fully stretched or contracted. This is approximately the angle where the muscle contracts the strongest so you can activate more muscle fibres in this position once the right weight is selected. For most weight training movements, the midrange position is the strongest range and can be utilised to activate more motor units. It stands to reason, then, that heavier weights can be used in this range and this range can be focused on. The stretch is the range of movement where the muscle is fully stretched. An example of a fully stretched position would be the outer range on a chest exercise such as the flyes, or the outer range on an exercise such as preacher curls for the bicep. This maximises the tension on the muscle tendon junction and can be used to strengthen this attachment and also the attachment from the tendon to the bone. It tends to be a weaker part of the movement and less weight is required to activate the muscle in this range. The contraction – this, in physio terms, is classed as the inner range part of the movement. So, for example, on the biceps, as you take the hand up towards the shoulder, it's the last 45 degrees or so of movement. For an exercise such as leg extensions for the quadriceps it would be the last few degrees towards lockout. This part of the range is useful when attempting to isolate certain muscle groups such as the long head of biceps. The long head of biceps works as a partial shoulder flexor so when the elbow is held high and that

68

inner range contraction part of the movement is utilised, the long head of the bicep contracts maximally. Similarly, for the quadriceps on the last few degrees of lockout, a muscle called vastus medialis obliquus is contracted and this helps to stabilise the knee from the inside. A well-known bodybuilder who was a two time Olympia winner, called Larry Scott, famous for his legendary biceps actually used this concept in the 60s before it had a name. He utilised this for his biceps. In more modern times, the ever popular barbell exercise called 21s, where you perform seven reps in the bottom half of the movement, the top half and then full range, is a prime example of angular training. It's a useful concept to incorporate into workouts but not to rely on it entirely.

Static Contraction Training

It's strange how bodybuilding mimics the fashion industry in many aspects, and this is just one of them. Static Contraction Training came back in fashion in the 1990s and most people didn't even realise that it had been also done in the 1930s.

Volume Training

In a similar vein, in the early 2000s and beyond, we go back to the 50s, back to volume training again. You could also consider the 1970s to be a volume training era. It's often related to the pump that is achieved through performing multiple sets.

Functional Training

The American Council on Exercise defines functional strength as performing work against resistance in such a manner that the improvements in strength directly enhance the performance of movement so that an individual's activities of daily living are easier to perform. Quite a mouthful. A simplified definition would be training that attempts to mimic the specific physiological demands of real life activities. Like most exercise

69

philosophies, there is some controversy over the term functional training. Mel C. Siff, PhD published a paper in the National Strength and Conditioning Association journal and said that, "functional training has become such a hot item that its proponents are creating the impression that all other approaches to sports training are wrong, unproductive, spurious, or ineffectual." Siff argues that the word functionality is highly subjective because it depends not only on the exercise itself but also on factors like:

- Characteristics of the athlete
- Reps
- Sets
- Manner of execution
- Phase of training
- Interaction with other training
- Current physical and mental state of the athlete

Regardless of the context in which we define functional training, clinical data from a multitude of sources clearly shows the effectiveness of functional training particularly for older adults. As we age, muscle mass and strength will decrease. The other thing that decreases is what we call proprioceptive capability. This means the subconscious knowledge of the position of joints in space. So this, in combination, means that older people struggle to perform tasks that involve resistance and coordination. Doing resistance exercises and movements that help you to become stronger, more flexible, more agile, and more coordinated are really useful for this group of patient. Functional strength training can be very sport specific and utilised well for athletes such as sprinters, rugby players, even tennis players and swimmers can benefit. Analysis of the characteristics of the athlete, the mechanics of the movement involved, i.e. the kinesiology, need to be taken into consideration. Generally speaking for the bodybuilder, however, functional strength training can be either beneficial or counterproductive. With the design of modern resistance machines now, strength curves can be established where the muscle contracts maximally throughout its full range. The advantage of these machines also is that it takes balance out of the equation, as it were. This means that less energy is wasted on stabilising muscles and muscles that help balance whilst the main prime movers are active. This allows for more concentration for the prime movers to create more muscle motor unit activity which can translate into better hypertrophy. However, I do believe that it's important to develop good core strength, balance and coordination using barbells and dumbbells. An experienced athlete can develop a groove of movement, which he can get into to maximise his response from his prime movers, i.e. the muscles that he primarily wants to train. It's good to help the beginner to develop this kind of coordination as well. I think the best designed workouts for the bodybuilder combine both free weights and the machines with a well-designed program. There are three areas where I do feel the bodybuilder can benefit. During the chapter on Therapy, we will go through three areas where I believe bodybuilders can benefit by improving their functional strength.

1. The deep abdominals (transversus abdominis and internal and external obliques)
2. Hip abductors and rotators
3. Scapular/shoulder stabilisers

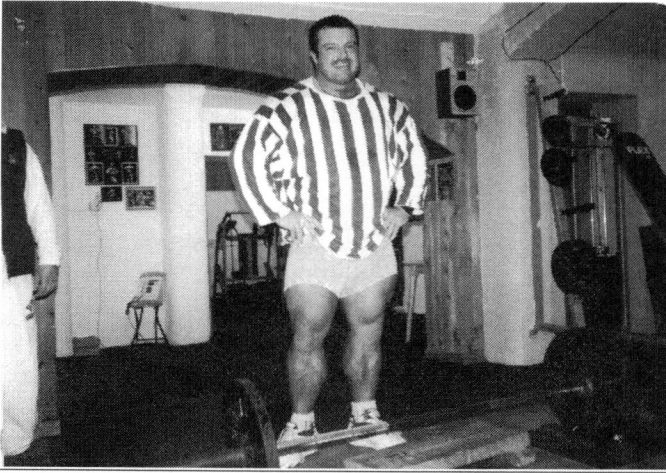

Myself, only just able to stand after a gruelling leg session with Doz at Dorian's Temple Gym in Birmingham during the 90's!

Occlusion Training

Blood flow restriction training (occlusion training) is making waves of late. It sounds new, it sounds scientific and some say it's revolutionary. It also smacks of artifice. It sounds like it was contrived by marketers to sell the latest round of magazines, pills and powders. So if you're sceptical, good, you should be. If something sounds too good to be true, it almost always is. You'll learn after reading this book that there really is no shortcut to building a strong, muscular body. There are right and wrong ways of going about it, but if you analyse all these methods of training, going right back, and apply a physiological approach to them, you'll be able to sort the wheat from the chaff, as it were, and devise for yourself the best program possible for hypertrophy. Blood flow restriction training involves restricting blood flow to a muscle group whilst training. The first thing they emphasise when advising people about

72

occlusion training is that it's not the goal to completely cut off the blood supply to a muscle. It's simply to slow down the rate at which blood returns from muscles to the heart. This causes blood to remain inside your muscles for longer than normal. Blood is the body's delivery system for oxygen, nutrients, glucose, hormones and other compounds needed to simply stay alive, let alone lift weights. Muscles need a regular, steady supply of blood to work. Your heart pumps blood to the muscles via the arteries which are large muscular walled, tube-like structures running throughout the body, that blood then is transported into smaller structures called arterioles and then eventually into capillaries where they deliver the nutrients they need to deliver to the muscle. Then, by way of venules and eventually veins, it takes the blood back to the heart. When you engage in resistance training, especially high rep ranges, the amount of blood going from your heart to the muscles outpaces the amount returning from your muscles to your heart and that's why you get a pump. The pump diminishes when you rest in between sets because arterial flow drops and blood is slowly evacuated from the engorged muscles. The point of blood flow restriction, or occlusion training, is to prolong this pump. This is accomplished by tying a band around the limb that you're training which allows blood to pump in but restricts the flow out. The theory behind maintaining blood within the muscle is that there are certain molecules within the blood that act as anabolic signals telling your body to increase muscle size and strength. If these molecules are maintained longer within the muscle, this trigger process allows a greater anabolic effect on the muscle cells than if the blood was being pumped out. It's also argued that cells expand and fill with fluid and nutrients when the muscle is engorged with blood. This is known as cellular swelling and this too acts as a signal for muscle growth. Studies have also shown that blood flow restriction training increases levels of MTOR and lowers Myostatin levels. This creates an environment in your body more conducive to muscle growth. These are the theories, but let's look at the facts that we know so far.

1. Although proponents of this method suggest that whilst blood flow leaving the muscle is restricted, the blood

73

flow entering the muscle is not restricted. This is not the case. Any kind of tourniquet device applied to a limb at the point where blood flow enters in the muscle will always restrict arterial blood to some degree.

2.   Oxygen flow will be restricted. Oxygen is needed for metabolic process to occur and glycolysis to occur in the muscle. After the muscle has been exposed to tension for more than 30 seconds, oxygen is required, this will lead to poorer contractions and less stimulus.

3.   Although MTOR levels may increase, and Myostatin levels may go down, this is also the case long term following heavy resistance exercise.

In conclusion, whilst I am not entirely against this form of training, I do believe that you could only use it as an adjunct and it shouldn't form the main framework of your workout.

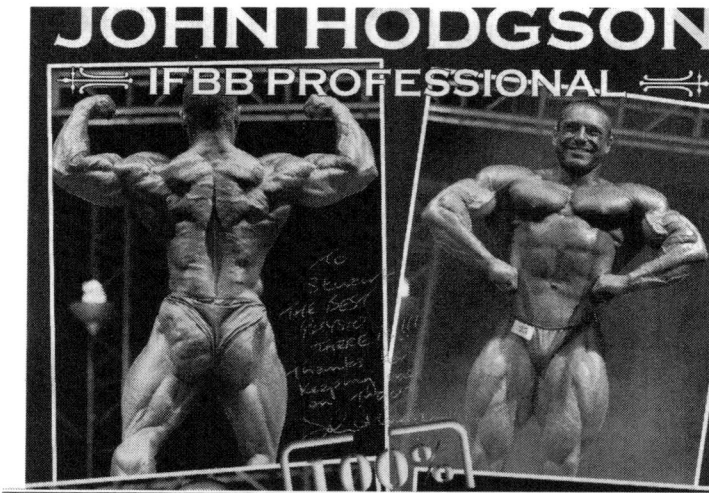

John Hodgson: With 3 EFBB British Titles and a Procard and Olympia qualification to his name, he is known for bringing a granite like physique to the table by using the High Intensity training techniques outlined in this book.

Chapter 5 – Bodybuilding Methods Throughout the Ages – Summary

1930s – Static Contraction

1950s – Volume Training

1960s – PHA Training
HIT Training
Periodisation

1970s – Bulgarian Method
Pre-exhaustion
Heavy Duty

1980s – Weider System
Super Slow
Holistic Training

1990s – Angular Training
Static Contraction Training

2000s – Volume Training
Functional Training
Occlusion Training

CHAPTER 6
THE IDEAL TRAINING PROTOCOL FOR MUSCLE GROWTH

I have no doubt that, as a discerning reader, as you were going through that last chapter about bodybuilding methods throughout the ages, you were having a chuckle to yourself because, as you learnt in previous chapters, especially Chapter One about Muscle Structure and Function, and Chapter Two about Energy Systems and Muscle Fibre Types, you recognised that a few of the training methods didn't exactly fit in with regard to the physiology of the muscle.

For example, if you apply logic, why would you ask a bodybuilder to do a volume training program? It's like asking a marathon runner to lift heavy weights. Also, when you compare the physiques of athletes that do volume training, as in marathon runners, long distance runners, even middle distance runners, their physiques don't compare to that of a sprinter or a weight lifter, or somebody who does low volume. As we know from athletes that develop the Slow Twitch red muscle fibres, their muscles can never enlarge as much as somebody who develops the Fast Twitch short duration white fibres. Having said that, there are some good take-home messages from each of the training methods that we have been through.

So now we're about to apply all the muscle physiology you've already learnt from the earlier chapters. If you look at the diagram entitled 'Training Protocol' we will go through each of the training methods in turn.

TRAINING PROTOCOL		
1 - FG (GLYCOLYTIC)		
SETS	**REPS**	**% 8RM**
1	15	25%
2	10	50%
3	6	75%
4 - PRIMER	1-2	80-100%
5 – WORKING SET	6-8	100%
TIME UNDER TENSION (TUT) 30 SECS		
TIME FOR 1 REP 4 SECS		

2 - FOG (OXIDATIVE - GLYCOLYTIC)		
SETS	**REPS**	**% 8RM**
1	15	25%
2	10	50%
3	6	75%
4 - PRIMER	1-2	80-100%
5 – WORKING SET	12	100%
TIME UNDER TENSION (TUT) 60 SECS		
TIME FOR 1 REP 5 SECS		

3 - ECCENTRIC		
SETS	**REPS**	**% 8RM**
1	15 (normal cadence)	25%
2	10 (normal cadence)	50%
3	6 (normal cadence)	75%
4 - PRIMER	1-2 slow negative	80-100%
5 – WORKING SET	6 slow negative	100%
TIME UNDER TENSION (TUT) 60 SECS		
TIME FOR 1 REP 10 SECS (7 secs negative, 3 secs positive)		

Number 1 is Glycolytic. The term glycolytic, as we've learnt earlier, refers to the Fast Twitch glycolytic white fibres that grow the most. These are the fibres that we need to predominantly train. As you can see from the table, the time under tension for these fibres is 30 seconds. If we give the time for each rep at four seconds, that is three seconds on the downward part of the movement, or the eccentric part, and then one second of explosive concentric to drive the weight out. So if the time under tension is 30 seconds, and the time for one rep is four seconds, that means the working set, when you're training to failure should be between six to eight repetitions.

Now, obviously, as a physiotherapist, I advocate a good stretching protocol before workouts and also before starting a body part. So we're assuming that you've stretched the muscle that you want to train. So now we move on to the first set. The first set is 15 repetitions. So you do 15 repetitions with 25 percent of your eight rep maximum. So the weight that you can do maximally for eight repetitions, we're using 25 percent for the first set. This should give you an easy 15 repetitions to do.

We can rest one to two minutes then, and then we perform set number two, this is for ten repetitions at 50 percent of your eight rep maximum weight. As we go up in weight, we rest a little bit longer so maybe two minutes before we do set number three, and this is for six repetitions at 75 percent of your one rep maximum. Now rest a good two to three minutes before attempting your primer set. As we've learnt earlier in the book, this primer set is really a means by which we maximally contract all the muscle fibres available to us by utilising as many motor units as we can but only for one to two repetitions so that we don't fatigue the muscle. So, basically, we're just firing the muscle up maximally before we do the working set. As you can see, I've given the percentage of the eight rep maximum at between 80 and 100 percent. In my experience, after having trained athletes, myself for many years, using this principle, and then also utilising it in my own workouts, I am moving closer to 100 percent for the primer set. The reason for this is, it will maximise even more motor unit recruitment. However, obviously, as you're using heavier weight, you've more chance of fatiguing the muscle. So I'm finding that we can rest for up to three minutes, possibly even longer for legs, before that priming system starts to shut down. This will make sure that we clear out all the lactic acid and that we reenergise the creatinephosphate system to give us all the driving potential for a maximal working set of six to eight reps then. So a good three minutes rest after the primer before you perform your working set.

In an ideal situation, where everything's working maximally and you can work to your ultimate failure, you should only need to do one working set. There will be some of you out there that are training on your own, without a training partner and it's sometimes difficult to get a spot. So in your situation, just to make sure that you really work the muscle to failure, I would possibly do two working sets but no more than this.

The second training method in our training protocol is oxidative glycolytic. It's working the FOG fibres. So if you remember, there are some white fibres that are kind of in between. These still hypertrophy and they tend to respond to slightly higher repetitions or, more correctly, a slightly longer time under tension. These fibres last for up to 60 seconds. What I like to do with this type of training is to take slightly longer to do repetitions, so we emphasise the eccentric, or the lowering part of the movement just that little bit longer. This is good for repair of the muscle tendon junction and allows the tendon to recover just that little bit quicker. So if you allow time for one repetition to be five seconds, and it's 60 seconds total time under tension, this allows for twelve repetitions for the working set. So we can apply the same principle with the warm up sets that we did before, except this time the percentages are of a percentage of the twelve repetition maximum. So the maximum weight you can do for twelve repetitions in your working set and you work on a percentage of that for the warm up sets. The same principle applies for the primer. I am erring more towards the hundred percent of the twelve rep maximum rather than the 80 percent to be more beneficial. As for rest periods in between sets, I would use the same rest periods that you did for the FG glycolytic training.

Finally, we move on to the eccentric training. The eccentric training is designed to activate the muscle contraction in a negative fashion. This actually causes more growth hormone production in the form of mechano growth factor or MGF as it is known. This is an isoform of insulin growth factor, or IGF, and is formed directly in the muscle as a result of this training. Another reason for doing this type of training is that it allows the tendon to recover and especially the muscle tendon junction. So where the tendon joins to the muscle there is a metabolic difference. The turnover of the muscle is much faster than the turnover of the tendon in metabolic time. This means that the muscle recovers much quicker than the tendon following a heavy workout. So it's useful to punctuate your training schedule with periods of eccentric training. As you'll see, the time under tension for the set is 60 seconds, the same as the FOG type training, but the time for one repetition is different. Each repetition lasts for ten seconds. That's seven seconds on the lowering part of the movement, or the negative part of the movement, and three seconds on the positive. This is clearly demonstrated on the DVD. As for the warm up sets, we do the first three sets with a normal cadence. So that would be a similar cadence to the FOG type training. The percentage of the weight used on these warm ups is the percentage of the six rep maximum. This is the six slow rep maximum. It's the slow negative maximum that you would use on this style of training. As you can see, the percentages are outlined on the right hand column. Only the primer is done as a slow negative repetition. This style of training can be applied to every exercise in your program. So now we've established these three different types of training style, glycolytic, oxidative glycolytic and eccentric, we need to incorporate them into your program.

If we look at the next table, called 'Cyclic Periodisation' we can see how to arrange these different styles in a format that maximises muscle hypertrophy but also allows for recovery.

CYCLIC PERIODISATION	
WEEK	STYLE OF TRAINING
1	GLYCOLYTIC TRAINING (FG FIBRES)
2	GLYCOLYTIC TRAINING
3	GLYCOLYTIC TRAINING
4	ECCENTRIC TRAINING
5	GLYCOLYTIC TRAINING
6	ECCENTRIC TRAINING
7	GLYCOLYTIC TRAINING
8	ECCENTRIC TRAINING
9	OXIDATIVE-GLYCOLYTIC TRAINING
10	GLYCOLYTIC TRAINING
11	PUSH/PULL SUPER SETS
12	WEEK OFF (STRETCHING ONLY)

This program is a twelve week cycle but this can be varied according to each person's needs. This is a typical example, this twelve week cycle, and it's something I would experiment with. Try this system first, but it's not set in stone and these weeks can be adjusted according to how you are progressing. Usually, at the start of a program like this, the first three weeks you tend to improve in strength and intensity almost exponentially. This being the case, it's good to run with it and as you improve each week go with the flow, as it were. However, a word of caution, it can lead you into a false sense of security and better bodybuilders than me have fallen at this hurdle. They've got so carried away with the weight gains, especially if they're on ergogenic aids, that they carry on. Sometimes early warning signs of tendon structure deformation are either missed or ignored. For example, in a compound press for the chest the weight goes up exponentially, and they keep going, and they keep going and then, eventually, something gives. This is the reason why I've given three weeks only for the really heavy duty glycolytic training before you intersperse with an eccentric week. This can benefit in two ways. The eccentric week can cause more growth factors to be released in the muscle, to maximise growth anyway. It can also help to prevent injury. It can help the tendon metabolism to keep up or at least catch up to that of the muscle. So I've put the first three weeks as glycolytic, the fourth week eccentric, and then back to glycolytic, then back to eccentric, alternating until we get to week nine.

Week nine we've introduced oxidative glycolytic. This also has the benefit of de-loading the muscle slightly but still loading the oxidative fibres maximally. One more glycolytic training follows this on the tenth week and then we go into week eleven. Week eleven employs something that we've already gone through in the training methods through the ages. You could apply any of the volume training methods just for this week. So you could utilise the Weider methods, super set methods, giant sets. I would generally encourage you to do a push/pull so you work the muscle antagonistically, so you work opposing muscle groups, and you could construct something up to a three, four, even up to a giant set program for each exercise. This would be like a giant weight training circuit training method. Obviously, this would diminish the weight you could use but at the same time improving oxygen uptake and also maintaining the capillary network for the muscles. This, believe it or not, is almost like a recuperative week for the repair of connective structures. So, basically, you are enhancing your blood flow to these structures without degrading them. Finally, week twelve is a complete week off, the only thing you should be doing on this week is

81

possibly a little bit of stretching and then you're ready to start week one, and start the cycle again. If you feel that you need more rest at week twelve, you could possibly take two weeks off then before you start the cycle again.

So, as you can see from this training protocol, we have employed a number of techniques from those that we've already studied. We've incorporated quite a lot of things and we've also incorporated everything we've learned from the physiology of the muscle. This is applying science to the method of bodybuilding.

I truly believe that this is the only way that you can maximise your results if you're like me, if you're a bodybuilder that responds to hard work and intense training, but you're not a genetic freak like some of the bodybuilders that we see at the top of the game. Believe me when I say that having trained with the best men in the sport, not all the top guys can adhere to this intense training method. Don't think that the guy with the biggest muscles trains the hardest, it might be that he's just more genetically gifted than you are, but it doesn't mean to say that you can't improve yourself and maximise your results.

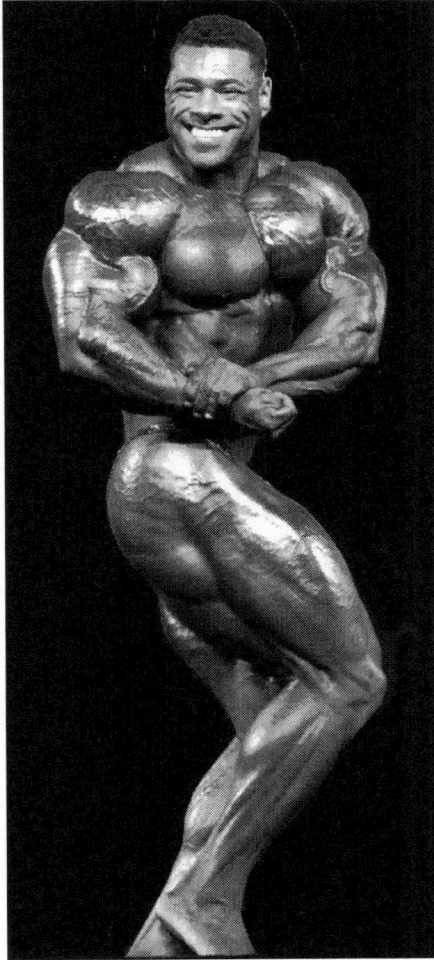

Nathan de Asha: Nathan is Britain's brightest hope at the Olympia contest. he recently won 2 Pro Shows and has had a 7th and 8th placing at the 2017/2018 Mr Olympia competitions! He is on the cusp of greatness and we are privileged to have assisted him to achieve this at Cosgrove's.

Chapter 6 The Ideal Training Protocol for Muscle Growth
SUMMARY

1) <u>FG Glycolytic Training</u> Starting at 25% of your 6-8 rep maximum, perform 10-15 reps for your first warmup. Then increase to 50% and do 10 reps. Third warm-up is 75% for 5-6 reps. Then primer set is done for 1-2 reps at the weight you will use for your set. Make sure you rest in between sets. At least 2-3 minutes after the primer before you start your working set.

2) <u>FOG (Oxidative/glycolytic) Training</u> The same procedure for the warm-ups as Glycolytic training , except it's a percentage of your 12 rep max rather than 6-8. Your working set should be aimed at 60 secs of Time under Tension or 12 reps. Still rest adequately between sets.

3) <u>Eccentric Training</u> Do your warm-ups the same as the other 2 methods with normal cadence and rest periods. Then perform the Primer as you would the working set. Use the same weight you will do on your working set but only do 1-2 reps with a 7 second lowering or slow negative. Then rest 2-3 minutes and attempt 6 slow negative reps to failure on the working set.

Use the Cyclic Periodisation Table to plan your schedule.

Chapter 7
Constructing a Training Program

From the previous chapter, we have the training protocol in place, and we've got the training cycle in place. Now we need to know how to construct the program to train each of the body parts and also when to train each of the body parts.

As you remember, in Chapter 5 we discovered many different training timetables or many different splits for how to split the body up. Whilst it must be said that it's very difficult to isolate each muscle group on its own, we do need to adhere to a certain means by which we split the body parts up so we don't overlap too much. Muscles tend to work in synergy, or tend to help one another in order to provide the movement. This is even more the case when doing functional strength training, i.e. strength training for a particular sport, such as rugby, involves using a series of muscles to perform the movement efficiently and effectively. This involves a chain of synergistic muscle contractions all in sync with one another to provide the accurate movement. Whilst this is beneficial specifically for that sport, it incorporates many muscles which are used for coordination and balance. As a bodybuilder, we need to consider this as being excessive use of energy which involves too much contraction of muscles not directly classed as the primer movers. In other words, sometimes in bodybuilding, it's good to take "balance" out of the equation.

Whilst some may consider exercise machines to be an ineffective means to gain strength and size, sometimes, when they are constructed with a degree of biomechanical efficiency, they can be very beneficial. Two people that looked into this in-depth were the bioengineer Arthur Jones and his associate, Ellington Darden MD. Between them, they forged the way, in the 1980s especially, with a range of machines called Nautilus. His son, Gary, took over in 1989 and formed Hammer Strength. He designed biomechanically sound weight training equipment which took balance out of the equation and maintained the strength curve that his father, Arthur, first developed with the 'D' cams. This equipment is very low friction, mimics the way the body wants to move and is very low maintenance. I can attest to the bearing systems lasting for 20 plus years.

Whilst these machines are top of the range, I would always prefer free weights over a poorly constructed machine. With free weights, the body can adapt to its own natural line of movement and although balance is involved with dumbbells and barbells, sometimes this natural line of movement can allow for maximum contraction of the primer movers. In bodybuilding terms, you can get a good groove of movement and once you're in the groove, you can really generate a lot of force of contraction. So in conclusion, with regard to selecting machines and free weight exercises, I would usually do a combination of both, providing the machines are either Nautilus, Hammer Strength or of similar high quality.

With regard to TABOO exercises, I tend to avoid;

- Lunges - they are so non-specific and require so much balance.
- Single arm dumbbell rowing - again, very non-specific and involve too much rotation.
- Full sit ups - they involve so much more than just the abdominals.
- Leg raises - for the same reason.
- Bench press – because it involves far too many muscle groups other than the chest, very non-specific.
- Any jerk pressing, cleans, clean and jerking.

However, the other two power lifts, the squat and the deadlift, although being classed as compound movements do engage large muscle groups with a large number of motorunit recruitment. With regard to the squat, I do now prefer, for bodybuilding purposes, to be done on a well-constructed squatting machine which takes balance out of the equation and allows the prime movers to function mainly. It also allows for specific foot positioning for quads or glute emphasis. With deadlifts, a massive motorunit recruitment is required in the

86

posterior chain muscles running down the back and also the quads. I would always use the deadlift to be periodically interspersed in your training schedule rather than being a constant feature.

Four Day Split Schedule

As you can see from the table, I've listed the days down on the left and then the body parts on the right.

Four Day Split Schedule	
Monday:	Chest, Triceps
Tuesday:	Back, Abdominals
Wednesday:	OFF
Thursday:	Legs
Friday:	Shoulders, Biceps

Optional fat burning at low intensities for 30-45 minutes after workout on all days except leg days.

No intense aerobics after workouts. This could be optional on days off but no more than 2-3 times per week and, ideally, short duration interval aerobics or preferably TABATA training only.

An alternative four day split could also be the same as above, except having a day off after legs and moving shoulder/biceps to Saturday.

I consider this to be the most ideal split schedule for this program of training. So we can see chest and triceps, essentially pushing muscles, are done on the Monday. Pulling muscles in the back, but also including the abdominals are done on the Tuesday. After two days of intensive training there, we need a day off, so that's the Wednesday. Then legs can be done on the

87

Thursday. You have the option really of either having Friday off and training shoulders and biceps on the Saturday, or doing shoulders and biceps on the Friday and having a complete weekend off before you start the cycle again.

You notice that chest and shoulders are separated because sometimes there is a degree of overlap with the pushing muscles in both chest and shoulders. Also biceps normally associated with back is separated to allow a more intense workout for the biceps when they would be fresher on the Friday with the ability to utilise more resistance. Sometimes biceps get fatigued too much on a back day.

You'll notice that for people that require a boost to their metabolism, or to try and lean up, optional fat burning can be done after the workout, or alternatively it could be done early morning when the blood sugar levels are low and you're more likely to initiate fat burning. This could be done for 30 to 45 minutes at a low intensity. So, for example, a steady speed on a stationary cycle where you are not getting too out of breath, you're still able to hold a conversation. Fat burning shouldn't be done on a leg day because you've already used up most of your glycogen reserves in the legs and you need to allow the glycogen supplies to be replenished to give enough energy for protein synthesis in these muscles. You should never incorporate intense aerobics after a weight training workout. You are already depleted of glycogen and this just compounds the issue. It can also affect hormone signalling. These could be done on optional days off but no more than two to three times per week. In bodybuilding terms, this type of intense aerobics should only be performed for 15 minutes and the main reason for doing it is to try and maintain capillary density in muscle tissue, so you're opening up the blood supply, you're maintaining a good blood supply to the muscles, and also a degree of fitness anaerobic/aerobic. TABATA style interval training involves very, very intense work for a short period of time, i.e. 20 seconds with a ten second break in between each burst of 20 seconds. This is repeated for eight times and then the session is finished.

If we look at the three day split schedule table now – this is not the ideal schedule, but for people with busy timetables, finding it difficult to fit four workouts in, this would be the ideal split.

Three Day Split Schedule	
Monday:	Chest, Shoulders, Triceps
Tuesday:	OFF
Wednesday:	Legs
Thursday:	OFF
Friday:	Back, Biceps, Abdominals
Saturday:	OFF
Sunday:	OFF

Optional fat burning at low intensities for 30 -45 minutes on days off may be considered.

Short duration aerobic/anaerobic training may be done as intense interval training for no longer than 15 mins and only for a maximum 3 x per week. TABATA training could be considered.

For people that have fast metabolisms and also recover quicker from intense exercise, then I would recommend this five day split.

```
┌─────────────────────────────────────────────┐
│            Five Day Split Schedule            │
│  ┌───────────────────────────────────────┐   │
│  │   Monday:          Chest              │   │
│  │                                       │   │
│  │   Tuesday:         Back               │   │
│  │                                       │   │
│  │   Wednesday:       OFF                │   │
│  │                                       │   │
│  │   Thursday:        Legs               │   │
│  │                                       │   │
│  │   Friday:          Arms               │   │
│  │                                       │   │
│  │   Saturday:        Shoulders          │   │
│  │                                       │   │
│  │   Sunday:          OFF                │   │
│  ├───────────────────────────────────────┤   │
│  │  The above split may suit the younger │   │
│  │  athlete with a faster metabolic      │   │
│  │  turnover, but an older athlete or    │   │
│  │  one who seems to be prone to injury  │   │
│  │  should switch to a three or four day │   │
│  │  split with periodic rest weeks every │   │
│  │  two months.                          │   │
│  └───────────────────────────────────────┘   │
└─────────────────────────────────────────────┘
```

As you can see, it still doesn't involve training LARGE muscle groups for more than two days consecutively. Always have a rest on the third day. This type of split could suit the younger athlete.

All these schedules are based on a seven day cycle. I find that as strength athletes get older and ligaments and tendons don't recover as quickly, it might be beneficial to maybe go on a four day split but extend the periods in between to work it on a ten day cycle rather than a seven day cycle. I find this is beneficial for training legs, for example. I found as I got older that my legs weren't fully recovered, tendon and connective tissue-wise, within seven days, and I needed to rest a further three days before I hit them heavy again. So doing legs once every ten days is a good idea for people in my age group and older.

Now we come to the choice of exercises. If we look at the table entitled 'Workout Exercises – A Typical Workout', what I've done here is laid out a workout I would give to a strength athlete wanting to body build on a four day split program. You can check out the style of each of these exercises on the DVD.

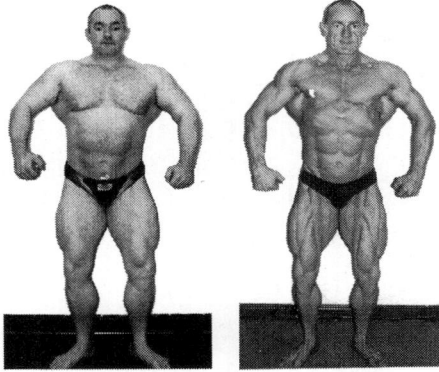

Colin Baron
1/ST SEPTEMBER 2000
WEIGHT 21 STONE
BODY FAT 24-5 %

Colin Baron
1/ST SEPTEMBER 2001
WEIGHT 14 STONE
BODY FAT 6-5%

Colin Baron: Colin transformed from 'smooth' powerlifter to competitive 'ripped' bodybuilder training at Cosgrove's Gym

WORKOUT EXERCISES (See DVD)
TYPICAL WORKOUT

CHEST	INCLINE PRESS (Barbell, Dumbbell or Smith Machine)
	FLAT OR INCLINE DUMBBELL FLYES
	SEATED PULLEY FLYES
	PEC-DECK (Inner Range squeeze/hold)
TRICEPS	OVERHEAD TRICEPS PRESS
	HORIZONTAL PULLEY/ROPE EXTENSIONS
	PUSHDOWNS
	SINGLE ARM REVERSE GRIP EXTENSIONS
BACK	PULLOVER MACHINE
	PULLDOWNS (Hammer Type Machine or Bar)
	ROW TO WAIST (Reverse Grip)
	HORIZONTAL ROW TO CHEST (over grip)
	HYPEREXTENSIONS or DEADLIFTS
ABDOMINALS	CRUNCHES & WEIGHT or AB MACHINE
	REVERSE PELVIC LIFTS (See DVD)
LEGS	LEG EXTENSIONS (Inner Range)
	V SQUAT or SMITH MACHINE SQUATS
	SISSY SQUATS (Feet together and back)
	LEG PRESS
	LYING HAMSTRING CURLS or CLOSED CHAIN HAMSTRING (See DVD)
	SINGLE LEG HAMSTRING CURLS (Preferably or SEATED CURLS if machine not available)
	ADDUCTOR MACHINE
	STANDING CALF RAISE or STRAIGHT LEG CALF PRESS (on leg press machine)
SHOULDERS	FRONT PRESS (Machine, Dumbbells, Barbell or Smith)
	SIDE LATERAL MACHINE
	INCLINE BENCH DUMBBELL LATERALS (See DVD)
	BENT OVER LATERALS
	SHRUGS (Dumbbells, Smith Machine or Calf Machine)
BICEPS	PREACHER TYPE CURL (Fixed Elbows)
	LYING PULLEY CURL TO FOREHEAD (See DVD) or BENT OVER BARBELL CURL TO FOREHEAD
	MID-POSITION ROPE PULLEY CURLS (See DVD)
	OPTIONAL: WRIST CURLS/WRIST EXTENSIONS USING PULLEY or DUMBBELLS

As it says in the title, it's just a typical workout. If I was to go through every possible exercise permutation for each muscle group, I would have a book the size of an encyclopaedia. For people wanting more ideas on different types of exercises, there are a number of examples on the DVD, but I would further recommend you read a book entitled, 'Keys to the Inner Universe,' by Bill Pearl. Bill Pearl was a top bodybuilder back in the 60s, highly respected, and this book is as thick as an encyclopaedia. I think the section on tricep exercises alone contains 300 different types of exercise permutations. What I aim to do going through this typical workout is to give you ideas for principles involved in selection of exercises.

Chest

If we start at the top, going through chest, what we need to do is analyse what type of muscle group the chest is. In anatomical terms, it's what we call a multipennate muscle. So the pectoral muscle is fan-like in shape. So it comes from a common origin, the sternum. This origin is very wide, covering a large area, and then it focuses in on an area of insertion on the top of the humerus. The muscle fibres come mainly in three distinct diagonals. You have the clavicular portion, which is the top part of the pectoral, which attaches to the clavicle. You've got the middle portion with horizontal fibres, and then you've got fibres coming at an angle from the lower sternum. These are the sternocostal fibres. If we think about the different angles of pull we need to work the chest from three different angles to try and maximise as much motor recruitment through each of these sections of the pectoral. When doing the incline press, you're mainly targeting the clavicular portion of fibres. This can be done using a barbell, dumbbell or a Smith machine. Whichever method you use, always make sure that the angle of the bench is no more than 25 degrees. The reason for this is to try and remove some of the emphasis on the anterior deltoid, or the front of the shoulder muscles, when doing this movement. The method of performing this exercise is shown on the DVD.

93

Next we want a flat type movement to target the middle fibres. I would recommend not to do a bench press movement as this is fairly non-specific when it comes to chest. Rather, do a flying type movement using dumbbells or pulleys. Next, target the sternocostal fibres. This is shown on the DVD as well, the seated pulley flyes, but with the back fixed. This allows for more concentration on the targeted area. Three exercises should suffice but to try and emphasise the inner range a pec-deck could be used.

Triceps

Moving on to triceps now, many gyms these days ignore the fact that the tricep muscle attaches over the shoulder joint as well as being attached to the elbow. As such, the largest head, being the long head, can only be fully contracted from a fully extended position with the elbow pointing to the ceiling. In our gym, we have an overhead tricep press machine which I personally think should be standardised across the industry. So this emphasises the largest long head, getting a full extension and full contraction, as I say, with the elbow pointing to the ceiling. This is demonstrated on the DVD. Then we could utilise a horizontal type extension, maybe using the ropes and a pulley, and then followed by push downs, which has been proven through MRI studies to emphasise mainly the lateral head. If you follow up with a fourth exercise to avoid too much overlap, I would recommend single arm reverse grip extensions. These are demonstrated on the DVD, and these would activate more the medial head of the tricep when done with this grip.

Back

When we look at the back anatomically, the back is similar to the chest in the fact that it's a multipennate muscle. Also incorporated into the back, you have many other muscles. Many of these muscles are associated with the scapula, or shoulder blade. These muscles attach to the shoulder blade at many different angles. Some can be highly developed such as middle trapezius and rhomboids and infraspinatus. Others are less apparent, such as serratus. The general rule of thumb with back training is to incorporate different angles of pull combined with different types of grip. As a rule of thumb I tend to suggest a high pull down to the chest, a low row into the waist and then a horizontal row to the chest. I also recommend varying the grip from over to mid and under, to incorporate many of these muscles, pulling at different angles. I tend to recommend four exercises for the upper back and one for the lower back. Arthur Jones developed the first pull over machine. This was designed to work the upper back in its entirety due to the large range of motion from a fully stretched position to a fully contracted position at the waist. A second generation version of this machine is shown on the DVD. This is similar to the one I trained with when I used to go to Dorian Yates Temple Gym. It was the mainstay exercise in Dorian's back program also. Following this, we can focus on a pull down movement from a fully extended position above to the chest. This could be done with a hammer type machine as shown on the DVD or using a lat bar. Make sure that you pull to the chest and not to behind the head. Then we need a row to the waist with a reverse grip ideally to emphasise the lower lats, and then this can be followed by a horizontal row to the chest.

As you notice on the DVD, the row to the waist is performed with the elbows down by the sides, and the horizontal row to the chest is performed with an over grip with the elbows high. This emphasises the rhomboids and the middle trapezius. That would complete the upper back workout. So we'd follow up now by working the lower back. This could be done with a deadlift, either stiff-legged or a full powerlifting style deadlift. Alternatively, for more isolation for the lower back, hyperextensions can be done. We have a specific machine for this in our gym. This can be demonstrated on the DVD. This can be weight-loaded also.

95

Abdominals

Now, with the abdominals, I tend to suggest working the upper and lower abs separately, trying to isolate these two groups as much as possible. I don't advocate doing a normal sit up, either with a straight or slightly bent knee. Neither do I advocate straight leg raises. Both these movements tend to over-activate the hip flexors and this takes away the focus of the abdominals. Also, with straight leg raises, this puts a shearing effect on the lower back, and anybody with a predisposition to mechanical low back pain will find this exercise eventually flares up their lower backs. So in order to isolate the upper abdominals, we need to restrict the range of movement. This is done by either a crunch style movement, where you are literally rotating around a pivot point at the lower sternal level. Don't attempt to go for a range beyond that crunch phase, otherwise then you will engage the hip flexors too much. For the lower abs, rather than straight leg lifting, we lift the legs already so that there is 90 degree flexion at the hip, and then we literally rock the pelvis up off the floor and hold. These are demonstrated on the DVD.

Legs

I always advocate legs to be done totally on the same day. So that is incorporating hamstrings also. There are many views on this but I run with the one relating to the hamstrings being partially worked when doing quads exercises, usually to help to stabilise in a squatting movement, and, therefore, if you try to do them on another day straight after legs you will tend to over-train them. So, in other words, if they're partially being worked then finishing them off completely and work them to maximum intensity while you can and then allow recovery to occur. When I used to train legs with Dorian Yates, we always had a 15 minute break after finished quads and this was done to stretch the quads to allow a full contraction of the hamstrings, and also to allow the hamstrings to relax somewhat. So you could maximise the weight/intensity. We're starting off with leg extensions. You have to consider that leg extensions primarily work as an open chain movement for the quads. They do, however, put a lot of stress on the cruciate ligaments. In view of this, it's important to do them in a really strict style without swinging and unnecessarily overloading with heavy weights. I always ask people to work on what we call the inner range. So that's the last 30 degrees of extension with a hold at the top, and place the feet at a ten to two position. This allows the muscle called VMO (vastus medialis obliquus) to work strongly. This is the main portion of the teardrop muscle and helps to stabilise the inside of the knee and is not worked adequately in any of the other quads movements. So that's why it's good to isolate it now. Don't bother too much with the rest of the movement of leg extensions as this is taken care of on the squat and leg press.

The next movement I advocate is a V-squat type movement with a squatting machine. If you don't have one of these leverage squatting machines then use a hack squat. Although I was a massive squat advocate, having a UK record for reps with 600lb for twelve reps, I don't now advocate using a barbell for bodybuilders. The squat machines take balance out of the equation and allow you to concentrate on feet positioning to work the prime movers that you want to develop. If you don't have a squat machine then use a Smith machine. Squats need to be controlled on the descent with a pause at the bottom, going full range, past 90 degrees, and driving outwards as explosively as you can. We then come to sissy squats which, with the feet positioned close together and the heels on a block or, as you see on the DVD, on a specially constructed platform, and these tend to emphasise the vastus lateralis for a good sweep on the quads. Good control is necessary as you see on the DVD. Then we use the leg press machine, again, with a good full range and control on the descent, and we also have an option of using band work on this exercise, as shown on the DVD also.

So after a period of rest and stretching the quads we come on to the hamstrings. Here, we do a lying hamstring curl with a contraction up to 90 degrees with a hold, then we follow this up with either single leg hamstring curls, preferably with a good full contraction and a hold at the top, going past 90 degrees this

97

time. Alternatively, you could use a seated machine, although I'm not a great advocator on the seated hamstring curls. You tend to be sitting on the muscle that you want to train and it can cause ischemia or a slight shutdown to the blood supply. If you look at the DVD we offer an alternative as well which could be done on alternate weeks, which is the close chain hamstrings. The beauty about this one is the hamstrings are contracting what we call reversed origin insertion. This means the hamstring contracts in the opposite manner to which it normally contracts for a normal leg curl. This exercise tends to get a really good pull and feel of DOMS near the hamstring attachment underneath the glutes.

Then we move on to adductors. Very often, the adductor muscles are missed out in many programs, bodybuilders will call these rather derogatorily a "lady's exercise". Nothing could be further from the truth. When you have a look at the biomechanics and the anatomy of the inside leg, it is comprised of four adductor muscles, two with large muscle bellies which need to be directly trained. It's no good saying, "Oh, well, I do a wide stance on the squats so I'll work my adductors." They would not be worked over maximum range with maximum intensity. So we need to localise this muscle group. As you can see on the DVD, these are done as heavy as possible with as strict a style as possible, with a hold on the inner range and a pause on the outer range whilst still under tension. Then we move on to calves. I always recommend a standing or straight legged calf movement followed by a bent knee calf movement in which you can position the toes differently. If you do a standing calf raise, either on a calf machine or on a squatting machine, lower the heels slowly until you almost reach rock bottom. Pause at the bottom of the movement and then explode out. It's important not to bounce at the bottom as this can irritate the Achilles tendon which wraps around the calcaneal bone. After this exercise then do a calf exercise with the knees slightly bent and fixed in that position, and the heels turned outwards and the toes turned in. This will emphasise the lateral head and also the soleus muscle. This can be done on a seated machine, as demonstrated on the DVD, or done on the leg press machine, fixing the knees with both hands in a flex position.

Shoulders

Again, with shoulders we just perform one pressing movement and we make it a front press rather than behind the neck press. Behind the neck press is very damaging for the supraspinatus and the rotator cuff and, also, over-stresses the anterior cap to the shoulder. The front press movement can be done using a machine, dumbbells, a barbell or the Smith machine. If using a barbell, drop to just slightly below chin level but don't come all the way down because of the undue stress it places on supraspinatus. I've known many strength athletes tear their supraspinatus by coming too low with a very heavy weight in a jerky motion. So, again, we control the weight downwards, pause at the bottom, killing momentum, and then exploding out to the top of the movement. It's optional, but you could 'not lock out' and keep the bar under tension. However, the deltoid still contracts right into a fully locked out position. So following this one pressing movement we then go into a side lateral movement. We demonstrate this on a side lateral machine on the DVD. As this is a fixed movement, but very isolating, you can find a position where your side deltoids are working effectively.

We can follow this up by an incline bench dumbbell laterals, also demonstrated on the DVD. As you can see, the line of pull is directly down through the side deltoids. Many people sit too high up or rotate the dumbbells laterally as they are lifting the dumbbells up. This throws the emphasis too much on the front deltoid. After the side deltoids, we work on the read deltoids by using a bent over lateral movement. It must be said that there is some overlap with this type of movement and working the rhomboids when doing back. This is another reason for placing your back routine far away from your shoulder routine in your program.

Finally, we come on to a shrugging movement. Now, I prefer to do shrugs more directly without having to grip dumbbells or a bar. This can be done on the calf machine. You have to be careful that you don't utilise your legs in this movement, that your legs stay static with your feet flat on the plate and you're just shrugging using the shoulder girdle. The head needs to be placed slightly forward so that you can offer a good range of movement and get a good hold at the top for a second or two, and killing momentum at the bottom and allowing the machine to stretch you. I find this more direct and effective. The only drawback to this exercise is that you are partially compressing the muscle that you want to train. Having said that, it is far more effective than holding dumbbells were the grip tends to go before the trapezius.

Biceps

With biceps, we look at the anatomy and we see that it's a two headed muscle, but one of the heads works over the shoulder. It also assists in shoulder flexion. So knowing this, we would always include a movement which either incorporates a degree of shoulder flexion or holds a shoulder flexed position to allow a full contraction of this lateral head. Having said that, we start off with a preacher movement, which focuses more on the lower bicep, and the thick inner head. Then we can perform a lying curl to the forehead or a bent over barbell curl to the forehead. Nautilus actually do a specific machine where the elbow is held in elevation with the shoulder in flexion, allowing a peak contraction to occur on the lateral head. We then try and concentrate on the brachialis muscle by doing a mid-position curl. In this curl we can either use a rope, and we can do it on a preacher machine, or we can do rope pulley curls. Always use a mid-position grip rather than a reverse grip, as a reverse grip will tend to put too much stress on the extensor tendon origin of the elbow, giving rise to tennis elbow conditions. I've put on the list of exercises that it's optional to do wrist curls and wrist extensions depending on whether you feel your forearms are lacking or not.

Four Day Split Schedule	
Monday:	Chest, Triceps
Tuesday:	Back, Abdominals
Wednesday:	OFF
Thursday:	Legs
Friday:	Shoulders, Biceps

Optional fat burning at low intensities for 30-45 minutes after workout on all days except leg days.

No intense aerobics after workouts. This could be optional on days off but no more than 2-3 times per week and, ideally, short duration interval aerobics or preferably TABATA training only.

An alternative four day split could also be the same as above, except having a day off after legs and moving shoulder/biceps to Saturday.

WORKOUT EXERCISES (See DVD)
TYPICAL WORKOUT

CHEST	INCLINE PRESS (Barbell, Dumbbell or Smith Machine)
	FLAT OR INCLINE DUMBBELL FLYES
	SEATED PULLEY FLYES
	PEC-DECK (Inner Range squeeze/hold)
TRICEPS	OVERHEAD TRICEPS PRESS
	HORIZONTAL PULLEY/ROPE EXTENSIONS
	PUSHDOWNS
	SINGLE ARM REVERSE GRIP EXTENSIONS
BACK	PULLOVER MACHINE
	PULLDOWNS (Hammer Type Machine or Bar)
	ROW TO WAIST (Reverse Grip)
	HORIZONTAL ROW TO CHEST (over grip)
	HYPEREXTENSIONS or DEADLIFTS
ABDOMINALS	CRUNCHES & WEIGHT or AB MACHINE
	REVERSE PELVIC LIFTS (See DVD)
LEGS	LEG EXTENSIONS (Inner Range)
	V SQUAT or SMITH MACHINE SQUATS
	SISSY SQUATS (Feet together and back)
	LEG PRESS
	LYING HAMSTRING CURLS or CLOSED CHAIN HAMSTRING (See DVD)
	SINGLE LEG HAMSTRING CURLS (Preferably or SEATED CURLS if machine not available)
	ADDUCTOR MACHINE
	STANDING CALF RAISE or STRAIGHT LEG CALF PRESS (on leg press machine)
SHOULDERS	FRONT PRESS (Machine, Dumbbells, Barbell or Smith)
	SIDE LATERAL MACHINE
	INCLINE BENCH DUMBBELL LATERALS (See DVD)
	BENT OVER LATERALS
	SHRUGS (Dumbbells, Smith Machine or Calf Machine)
BICEPS	PREACHER TYPE CURL (Fixed Elbows)
	LYING PULLEY CURL TO FOREHEAD (See DVD) or BENT OVER BARBELL CURL TO FOREHEAD
	MID-POSITION ROPE PULLEY CURLS (See DVD)
	OPTIONAL: WRIST CURLS/WRIST EXTENSIONS USING PULLEY or DUMBBELLS

Exercise Style

Each of the exercises needs to be done in a controlled manner, pausing at the end of each range, making sure that you kill momentum so it can't assist you in any way. The movement should be lowered slowly in a controlled manner and then exploded out from the bottom part of the movement, and then held at the top for a second before lowering again. All the exercises on this workout sheet can be performed in this manner.

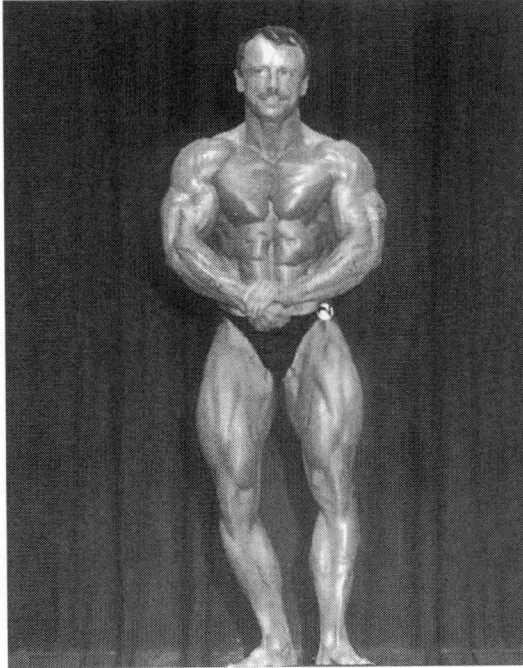

Kerry Kayes: One of the most famous and popular Bodybuilding and Boxing coaches. He transformed conditioning and nutrition for the world of Professional Boxing during the Hatton Era. His company CNP used to supply nutritional products to and advise the Sky British Cycling Team. he achieved this condition, winning the Senior British Title.

Chapter 8
What Prevents a Muscle from Responding

1) POOR NUTRITION
2) INADEQUATE FLUID INTAKE
3) OVERTRAINING (lack of Periodisation)
4) CONNECTIVE TISSUE STRESS
5) HORMONAL STRESS AND IMBALANCE
6) POOR SLEEP PATTERN

All the above factors can affect how a muscle responds to training. They all, also, tend to influence one another and therefore all need to be at optimum level for muscle development to succeed.

We will start with:

1)   POOR NUTRITION

a) MACRONUTRITION (ie. Protein,Fats,Carbohydrates)

Protein

Protein Level and Quality: Protein as we know is the main constituent of cells. It is broken down into amino acids by digestive enzymes in the stomach and small intestine. There are 9 Essential amino acids that need to be taken into the body from foods in order for the body to manufacture all the correct non essential amino acids to synthesise new proteins to be incorporated into the cells. If all 9 are not present in the protein being eaten, it can be classed as a poor quality protein.

We also need to take into consideration the digestibility of the protein. Some people are unable to properly or speedily digest the protein to derive its nutrition. Some proteins are naturally harder to digest, and also through age, our ability to digest proteins decreases. These things need to be taken into account when assessing the quality of a protein.

Within the 9 essential amino acids are 3 Branch Chain Amino acids (Valine, Leucine and Iso-leucine). These Branch Chain Amino acids (BCAA's) are cited in many studies as being of great importance in protein synthesis , especially in the recovery of muscle damage after intense resistance training. It would therefore be logical to find a good protein source that provides all 9 amino's including adequate BCAA's. Also, that it is adequately digested and utilised. Taking these things into consideration, the value of protein needs to be given a numerical number. Most people use the NPU (Net Protein Utilisation) score to rate the protein. In light of this, the following table lists some of these foods:

FOOD PROTEIN SOURCE	NPU VALUE
WHEY PROTEIN	92
WHOLE EGG	87
COWS MILK	81
FISH	80
CHICKEN	73
BEEF	73
SOY BEANS	67

As you can see, whey protein has the highest NPU of 92 % and therefore has the best quality of amino acids in a usable form. The only problem here is that it is digested and utilised so quickly, that if the body doesn't need all of it at that time, some will be oxidised for energy rather than be used to build more cell proteins!!

In 1991, a new scale was introduced by the Food and Agricultural organisation of the WHO (World Health Organisation). This is the current Internationally approved scale for Protein Quality Assessment. It is the PDCAAS (Protein Digestibility Corrected Amino acid Score). This takes into consideration the digestibility as well as the usability of the protein. It does, however flag up similar values to the NPU scale. As you can gather, animal protein tends to rate much higher on these tables than do vegetable proteins, having a higher biological value and digestibility. This is not to say that vegetarian proteins are no good, it's just that the right blend of pulses and vegetables has to be taken to get near to the biological value of animal proteins. Soy is widely accepted as one of the more complete sources of plant protein and therefore vegetarians are encouraged to consume soy-based proteins on a regular basis.

The best way to obtain your amino acid requirement daily is to eat a balance of animal and plant based proteins regularly. Whilst animal based proteins may have a better biological value, massive ingestion is associated with chronic disease such as colonic and digestive tract disorders. Vegetarian diets do tend to eliminate a predisposition to these diseases probably due to the fact that they contain a richer supply of antioxidants and phytochemicals to battle against free radical toxins and assisting the body's immune system.

So how much protein does a strength athlete need? Current research tends to suggest that a strength athlete needs 1.6 to 2 g of protein per kg of bodyweight. This assumes that the athlete is in a relatively lean off season condition (i.e. less than 12% bodyfat). This seems to correlate well with the extensive studies done by the Colgate Institute in California in the 1980's which studied the BUN (Blood Urinary Nitrogen) levels of athletes of all types and of varying levels of intensity in their training. Levels for females were approximately 2/3 that of the males, mainly due to higher natural bodyfat levels.

Carbohydrates

The general recommended levels of carbohydrates for strength athletes of high intensity is from 4-10 g per kg bodyweight in order to maintain a protein sparing, glycogen replenished state. The current trend in bodybuilding is to utilise a ketogenic type diet in order to lean the physique, whilst maintaining muscle mass. This is nothing new and was the type of diet used by bodybuilders in the 1980's to lean up for a competition. Indeed it was the typical diet I used to use for the first 5 years of competitions, until, of course, I eventually figured out how detrimental it was!! It involves starving the body of carbohydrates, whilst increasing protein and fat levels. The theory behind this is to force the body to utilise ketones as an energy source from the incomplete breakdown of fats in the liver and to prevent the release of insulin which has a tendency to deposit fat stores. This also encourages the body to use fatty acids from fat stores as energy.

Under normal conditions, fatty acids from fat stores are converted to glucose in the liver which is then transported to the cells to be used as energy (ATP) or stored as glycogen in the muscles. So this is the normal way of burning fat for energy. But in the case of starvation of the body from carbohydrates and very low insulin levels, the conversion in the liver switches to produce ketones. Now ketones can only be used by cells that contain mitochondria (the cells energy governor) such as nerve tissue, muscles and the brain. This is an amazing design to prevent central nervous system shutdown in times of starvation of its normal energy source. This system of energy production was only designed to be used for short periods of time during food shortage. As such, muscle breakdown is only prevented for the first couple of weeks, after which the muscle starts to be cannibalised as energy due to the shortage of carbs. The muscle is broken down to amino acids to try to step up energy supply to meet demand. These amino acids are converted to glucose (gluconeogenesis) the body's much preferred energy source! Advocates of the ketogenic diet argue that if you take enough BCAA's (Branch Chain Amino Acids) in, this will act as a strong protein synthesis driver to combat muscle wastage. What they fail to recognise is the amount of energy required to incorporate proteins into cells is far greater than that which is able to be supplied by this less efficient system. Net loss will always overcome net gain! Muscle protein synthesis requires the RNA messenger transcript system to utilise massive amounts of energy at one go, only possible from a massive glucose supply from carbohydrate sources. Trying to put on muscle whilst on a ketogenic diet is like stepping on the gas and applying the brakes at the same time!! I always say to bodybuilders on a keto diet,

107

just try upping your carbs and check yourself in the mirror over the next few days and you will see a transformation for the better!! There is no way you can move your maximum poundages and train to an adequate intensity on this diet! I know, because in the early days, I did this regularly precontest and used to mourn as I saw my poundages getting less and less. Only when I started to up my carbs precontest was I able to maintain my size and strength.

I remember when it first hit home! I was weighing 210lbs in the off season as a novice bodybuilder, with a body fat of 10%. This should have had me going on stage in competition at about 190lb. Instead, after a precontest keto diet, I went on at 165 lb. Granted, I was ripped, but at what expense!! I looked like a shadow of myself!! 25lb of muscle sacrificed!!

Fats

By this, I mean the Essential fatty acids. The body can synthesize the fats it needs from the diet. However 2 essential fatty acids that can't be synthesised are OMEGA 3 and OMEGA 6 fatty acids. These are found in foods such as primrose oil and in fish oils. They are also found in nuts and grain products. You don't need to consume fats in great quantities to acquire these essential fatty acids as long as you get the right combination of fats. The European SCF (Scientific Committee on Food) established total requirements for females of 6g of essential fatty acids per day (5g Omega 6 ,1g omega 3), and for males, 8 g (6.4g omega 6, and 1.6g omega 3) These fatty acids are necessary for the absorption, transport and utilisation of the fat soluble vitamins A, D, E and K. Studies have also shown that they can help prevent muscle breakdown. They help to produce prostoglandin E1 which is involved in growth hormone release. It must also be said at this point, that whilst the NHS is hellbent on reducing every man and his dog's cholesterol levels by indiscriminate use of STATINS, they fail to inform people how adequate cholesterol intake and manufacture is necessary to produce all types of hormones for health regulation of body homeostasis! In other words low level of Total cholesterol is far worse for the body than a high one. After careful analysis of the original studies for the link between high cholesterol and Heart disease, this link turns out to be a very tenuous one at best! (see the book ' The Great Cholesterol Con' by Dr Malcolm Kendrick) These essential fatty acids also improve insulin sensitivity, decrease inflammation and improve cardiovascular health. They also help to form cell membranes when they combine with amino acids to form lipoproteins.

b) MICRONUTRITION

By micronutrition, we mean adequate supply of Vitamins, Minerals, trace elements and antioxidants in the diet.

Vitamins

Vitamins A, D, E and K are all fat soluble vitamins and are stored in the liver and fat tissue until needed. They have a multitude of functions including maintenance of the matrix in bone and normal muscle function. Vitamin K allows your blood to clot, but is also involved in making proteins for muscle, bone and other tissues. Foods high in these vitamins are:

Kale, Spinach, Green Beans, Turnips, Lettuce, Parsley, Brussels Sprouts, Broccoli, Asparagus, Carrots, Squash, Sweet Potato, Liver, Milk and Cheese.

Vitamins B complex and C: These are water soluble vitamins and are therefore not stored in the body and should ideally be consumed regularly. They can easily be destroyed by heat or air, eg lost in cooking by boiling the foods and throwing the water away!   Most of the B complex vitamins are used for nerves, nerve conduction, energy metabolism and the digestive system.

Vitamin C is also called Ascorbic acid and is a powerful antioxidant in the body. It is also needed for collagen formation, an essential constituent of tendons and ligaments. It also assists the immune system in fighting disease.
B complex and Vitamin C are found in fruit (especially citrus), vegetables and grain products.

Minerals and Trace elements:

Like vitamins, these are found in foods. These are all required for growth and function and to keep the chemical reactions in the body in balance (Homeostasis). The Macrominerals are the ones your body needs in larger amounts. These are: Calcium, Phosphorus, Magnesium, Sodium, Potassium and Chloride.

The Microminerals or Trace elements are the ones your body needs in smaller amounts ie: Zinc, Iron, Copper, Iodine, Fluoride, Selenium.

Calcium, Magnesium, Phosphorus and Fluoride are all needed for bone and teeth growth and maintenance and also to help maintain a good nervous system. Calcium, Magnesium, Iron, Potassium and Sodium are all needed for normal muscle function. Sodium, Potassium and Chloride are all needed to maintain normal cellular water balance. Iodine is used to maintain normal metabolism (the Thyroid gland). Copper and Iron are used for red blood cell formation and delivery of oxygen to tissues. Zinc is needed for healthy skin and immune system helping wound healing and also for Testosterone production.

Antioxidants:

Under normal conditions, the body utilises the oxygen pathway cleanly to produce energy. However the pathway to energy production can be 'dirty' producing damaging substances known as 'free radicals'. These 'free radicals' are very damaging to cells, acting like metabolic shrapnel. They have consistently been linked to cells becoming cancerous. These free radicals can be 'mopped up' and removed by the antioxidants utilised by the body to protect itself from cellular damage. The 4 main powerful antioxidants are: Vitamin C, Vitamin E, Selenium and Co-Enzyme Q10.   Vitamin C, E and selenium are all derived from outside food sources. The body can manufacture its own Co-Enzyme Q10 for energy production. However, most of this is used up maintaining the bodies metabolism and

110

requires extra outside sources for it to be used as an antioxidant. People who train intensely use their Q10 up very quickly. Its production also declines with age, so it is essential that outside supplementation is given. People who use statins need an extra supply.

Other useful powerful antioxidants are Green Tea and Pycnogenol. The best Superfoods to supply these antioxidants are: Gogi Berries, Blueberries, Dark chocolate, Beans, Pecans, Artichokes, Elderberries, Kidney Beans, Cranberries.

2) INADEQUATE FLUID INTAKE

Not drinking enough either prior to or in the gym is a sure way to underperform. Signs of dehydration are as follows;

- Increased thirst
- Feeling dizzy or faint
- Lack of sweat
- Dark,strong urine
- Blurred vision
- Sunken eyes
- Rapid heart rate and breathing
- Lack of energy
- Muscle cramps

Water may seem like a simple molecule, but the fact that these 2 gases together exist as a liquid is nothing short of a miracle at all! It also performs miracles in the body with its untold chemical processes! If the average human did without water, he or she would die within a few days! But how much water does a human need per day? It all depends on body size, muscle mass, metabolism and activity levels. The WHO (world health organisation) recommends 2.7 litres for women and 3.7 litres for men per day, with 25% of it coming from food. So this would mean that 2 litres of water would have to be taken in drink form for women per day and 3 litres for men. People that drink high caffeine drinks such as coffee, tea and coke would also be negating their water intake somewhat due to the stimulatory effect to the metabolism, utilising more water for increased chemical reactions in the body. As a rough guide, only half the volume of a high caffeine drink could be classed as water intake. eg 500ml of coke is only equivalent to a water intake of 250ml. When we come to strength athletes with a higher proportion of muscle and therefore glycogen storing capacity, they may require up to twice the average intake of water. Every gram of carbohydrate stored as glycogen holds 3 grams of water in the muscle cell. Bodybuilders carbing up for a competition require a massive increased water intake. If he takes in 1000g carbohydrates, he will need at least 3 litres of water on top of his normal intake! It is important to take in this water on a regular basis. Don't forget, muscle is composed of 70% water , so don't lapse on your intake!

3) OVERTRAINING

Rest Days   The whole of the fitness industry has fallen back into the line of reasoning that 'more is better'!! If you want to increase the size of your arms and you are training them twice a week, why not increase that to three times or even four times a week to improve even more!! Rest days are a waste of time, when that time could be more productively spent in the gym!! This is the philosophy that pervades even the bodybuilding fraternity today!! So what have we learnt?? It's so difficult to get through to some athletes embarked on this spiral of overtraining that the interspersing of rest days would actually benefit their performance level!!

When you train hard in the gym, the release of 'feel good' chemicals such as adrenalin, endomorphins and dymorphins gives you a 'high', similar to (but healthier than) some recreational narcotics. As a result of this, some people become literally addicted to exercise, similar to drug addiction. This can be very detrimental to the body, not only in long term connective tissue damage, but also to the immune system and the stress controlling system.

However, from muscle physiology studies, we know how long it takes for muscle tissue to recover from intense resistance work!

Even if you schedule a really good split program, working antagonistic muscle groups e.g. push/pull type split, to allow one to rest as you train the other, its still very difficult to rest any muscle group whilst training in this fashion. Therefore, it is very important to incorporate a TOTAL rest day into your routine. This means no other activities for these muscle groups during that day! This allows the body to regain an anabolic status, over riding catabolism. This allows more protein synthesis to occur in the muscle to allow it to repair and grow. It should also be mentioned here, whilst we are talking about rest periods to also consider the rest periods between sets when performing an exercise. Very often with personal training programs these days , trainers and athletes alike seem to think you have to be out of breath all the time whilst training and that little or no rest between exercises should be employed to get the best results. As such weight training programs are getting more like circuit training programs. Whilst an overall modicum of strength and fitness may be achieved, it is not the best way to maximize muscle hypertrophy and strength! As we have spoken about already, if you do not rest adequately in between sets (i.e. 2-3 mins.), then you cannot recharge the creatine energy system which gives you explosive power output and also cannot mop up and reconvert lactate from the muscle.

Volume

With the current trend of going back to the '70's style of VOLUME TRAINING, most people do far too many sets per exercise. As we have discussed, its all about maximizing the greatest amount of tension in the muscle over a required amount of time! If we use the analogy of a joiner striking a nail into a piece of wood, once he has hit the nail so it is flush with the wood, does he then continue to strike it?? No! Because if he did, it would damage the wood and probably the nail as well! Its the same with the muscle you intend to grow and strengthen, once you have maximised its tension under time, then move on to the next exercise, don't keep hammering it!! This means in an ideal situation, with maximum concentration and a strong focus on MIND/MUSCLE connection, only ONE working set is

113

required. All the preceding warm up sets are preparatory sets, preparing the muscle for that 'all out' one set to failure!

Cardio

Sometimes we get athletes coming in who want to gain muscle, but also be supremely fit cardiovascularly as well. Whilst there is a degree of compromise allowed in this regard, I usually ask them, 'Do you want to excel as an endurance athlete or a strength athlete?' If they are strength training for a particular sport such as Rugby or Boxing, I usually ask them 'How long does the muscle have to work for at a high level of intensity?' For example, with Boxers, they work at high intensity for no longer than a 2-3 minute round, so I would never give them High Intensity for much longer than this timeframe. Similarly, for Bodybuilders to maximise the right muscle fibres, they should not be working at maximum intensity for longer than 1 minute.

I usually recommend TABATA style training for maximum anaerobic/aerobic threshold training as it maximises lactate and oxygen uptake training in one fell swoop! It also doesn't eat away at muscle mass like a moderate intensity long drawn out aerobic session lasting 20 mins to over an hour or more! TABATA was designed by a Japanese Exercise Physiologist who determined that a high level of cardiovascular efficiency can be achieved by doing high intensity, explosive short bursts of activity for a short period of time, followed by short rest periods. For example, on a stationary bike, after warming up for a minute or two, on a high resistance setting perform a short maximal burst of speed for 20 secs. Try to achieve in excess of 120 RPM. Then immediately drop back to 70RPM on a light resistance for 10secs, then repeat the cycle again until you have completed 8 cycles. On paper, this looks easy, but trust me, it will literally be the hardest aerobic activity you will ever do!. In fact, unless you are in amazing cardiac condition, you will not complete 8 cycles unless you drop intensity or extend your rest periods to 20 secs or more. It needs to be built up slowly! Because this TABATA is only done a maximum of 3 times weekly and because it is only for short periods, glycogen depletion and muscle atrophy are less likely to occur. It is one way a bodybuilder can keep a high cardiovascular efficiency. The other benefit to this training is it helps to improve capillary density in muscles, helping their circulation and also it helps clearance of Lactate or Lactic acid from the muscle faster for a quicker recovery time. Any longer periods of aerobic exercise should be done at an 'anaerobic pace', ie much less intensity so fatty acids can be burned instead of the need for oxygen from carbohydrates.

Periodisation

Periodisation, when applied to Bodybuilding means the cycling of various aspects of the training schedule. It could mean variation of any number of factors, such as exercise volume, intensity, time under tension, exercise selection, order, rep range and speed, rest intervals etc. The main aim is to maximise strength and muscle hypertrophy whilst at the same time preventing plateaus and injury and other catabolic effects of over training. These cycles could be classed as a MESOCYCLE of 6 to 12 weeks followed by a rest week. Then MICROCYCLES of various training methods could be applied within the main mesocycle. This prevents stagnation of muscle development, but also takes into consideration the metabolism of different tissues such as tendons, fascia and ligaments.

4) CONNECTIVE TISSUE STRESS

Quite often in my profession as a Strength Physio, I come across too many athletes who unnecessarily tear pectorals, biceps, triceps, lats etc. When I quiz them carefully about conditions leading up to their injury, it becomes apparent that they were repetitively overloading the muscle tendon junction and not allowing it to repair. Very often it was disclosed that the athlete was taking Anabolic Steroids or some other effective SARM or ergogenic aid. Usually as well, athletes suddenly embark on a course like this after either weeks of layoff or lazy training and suddenly load their bodies. They also tend to go with the flow and continue HEAVY, HEAVY, HEAVY glycolytic style training whilst their strength goes through the roof. The trouble is, tendons and ligaments cannot keep up with

115

vascular tissue like muscle metabolically speaking and so something has to give!! Very often it is at the point where the muscle blends in with the tendon and they end up with a muscle slide (see the next chapter). Sometimes the tendon may avulse or tear completely from the bone. Up till recently, surgeons used to blame steroids directly for causing weakness in the tendon. This doesn't stack up physiologically as anabolic steroids improve anabolism i.e. build tissues up! It is corticosteroids which are catabolic in their action. The degradation in the tendon comes from overuse and under-recovery.

In order to alleviate this connective tissue stress, slow negative training could have been introduced inbetween the heavy glycolytic training to allow the collagen to repair in the tendon and allow it to catch up metabolically to the muscle again. So this highlights the importance of varying the training program week by week. When we train the muscle intensely, it literally damages the fascia and microfibrils. As a result of this, an inflammatory reaction is set up to heal these tissues. If retraining of this affected muscle is repeated too early, without giving enough time to repair and recover, then damage can occur, which then elicits a 'Stress Response' which may affect the whole body.

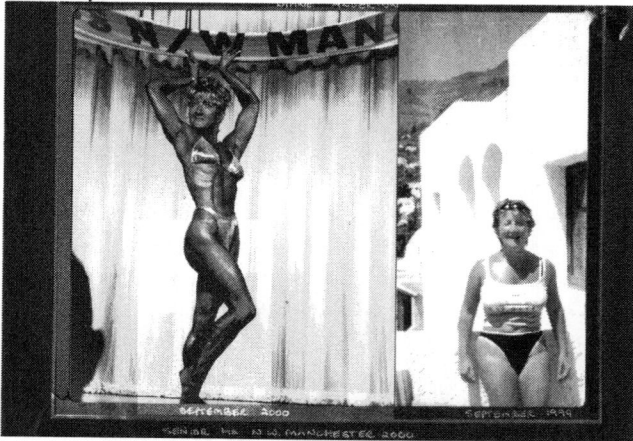

Diane Anderton: This is an amazing transformation in 12 months. She put forth a monumental effort to get in this shape training at Cosgrove's Gym. With our advice, she won Senior Miss Manchester 1999!

```
                    ┌──────► STRESS ◄──────────┐
                    │           │              │
                    │  Fatigue of vasomotor nerve cells
                    │           │              │
                    │  Relaxation of blood vessel walls
                    │           │              │
                    │   Slower rate of blood flow ──┐
                    │           │              │    │
                    │      Shrinkage of fascia ──┐  │
                    │      (Postural changes)    │  │
                    │           │              │  │
                    │      Weakening of muscles │  │
                    │           │              │  │
                    │    Biomechanical dysfunction │  │
                    │           │          │   │  │
         BIOMECHANICAL PAIN        ANOXIC PAIN
```

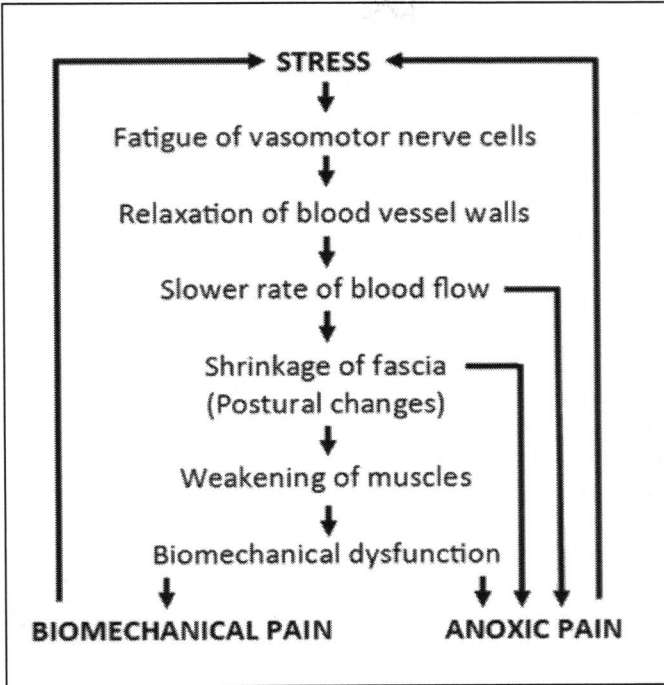

So as you can see from this chart, our bodies have a certain pattern they keep to when put under enough stress so as not to go beyond the limits of control. This stress table can be applied to other forms of stress apart from physical. It could be mental, energetic or emotional stress. If this applied stress goes beyond the body's threshold to cope, it will begin to damage the body. The body has a fantastic capacity to compensate, but once that limit has been breached, it will be exposed and it will begin to wear. Changes take place firstly on an energetic basis and then a physiological one.

One of the most common complaints we are confronted with as physio's is Repetitive Strain Injury or RSI. Now if we take a closer look at all the strength athlete injuries we see, we could probably say that 85% of them are a form of RSI. Also, the common reasoning that all RSI's are as a result of intense physical activity is a fallacy! . Even sitting on a chair for hours on end is a form of RSI! Tissues may be held in a fixed position for

117

long periods. This on its own is a form of overload! So any form of static over demand on a group of muscles designed for movement, where the muscles are held in a semi-fixed tone for long periods can cause stress on the VASO-MOTOR NERVE CELLS which cause disruption to the blood flow to these muscles. This means these nerve cells have to work extra hard to deliver adequate blood to these areas. This over fatigues these nerve cells. This leads to anoxic fatigue of the muscles, shrinkage of the fascia covering the muscle and pain. Repetitive stress on a muscle without allowing its normal recovery cycle to occur is a form of RSI. As you can see from the 'Stress Response Table', everything seems to revolve around adequate (or not as the case may be) blood flow to muscles. This is called Haemodynamics. The Chinese have been reporting this for hundreds of years and use acupuncture to restore blood flow or haemodynamics to tissues. As you can see from the table, it can be self-perpetuating, i.e. If blood flow is restricted to the muscle, this causes the fascia round the muscle to shrink, causing less oxygen to be transmitted to muscle cells, causing loss of function, causing more tension and stress on the nerve cells and so on!

The take home messages here are clear: 1) It is so important to rest adequately between workouts, 2) To rest adequately between sets, 3) To stretch well and also wherever possible 4) To find a therapist who does fascial and Active Release techniques to free the fascia to improve blood flow.

5) HORMONE IMBALANCE

Cortisol This a hormone secreted by the adrenal glands. Unlike Testosterone and Growth Hormone, Cortisol has Catabolic functions in muscle. It tends to break things down rather than build them up. In contrast, Testosterone and growth Hormone are anabolic and tend to build up the muscle tissue. A prime mechanism in the body whilst under stress is a rapid release of energy. Cortisol assists in this mechanism in the liver called GLUCONEOGENESIS. This involves converting non-carbohydrate nutrients into glucose in the liver. These could be amino-acids and fatty acids. Under the influence of Cortisol, Gluconeogenesis in the liver increases sixfold under stressful situations. Cortisol can mobilise amino acids directly from muscle tissue in order to produce this energy. This is the familiar Catabolic effect of muscle teardown.

Cortisol also affects carbohydrate metabolism by affecting the rate of glucose usage by the cell. It depresses glucose transport into cells, thereby decreasing glucose sensitivity. It also decreases muscle protein synthesis as it doesn't have the energy to perform it adequately.

Cortisol can temporarily increase ketone production from fat. Although ketones exert an anti-catabolic effect on muscle proteins, this is only the case for a couple of weeks or so on a ketogenic diet. Then the potent effect of cortisol far out weighs this in terms of catabolism and muscle tear down. This one major consideration to be aware of when embarking on a Ketogenic Diet. Any kind of muscle preservation will only last 2 weeks maximum, before catabolism and cannibalism of muscle tissue takes place. Another factor is that the rate of gluconeogenesis cannot keep up with glycogen usage, especially trying to train intensely with heavy poundages . Sooner or later, energy levels and therefore intensity will drop, giving less stimulus for protein synthesis.

Another effect of cortisol is its potent anti-inflammatory action, which is beneficial in stressful situations. When you have a large stress response elicited in the body, there is a large, initial catabolic effect. However, good periodisation can have a good compensatory effect. Exercise itself, whilst initially stimulating cortisol through the stress response, has a much greater compensatory effect on the muscle. Also, more conditioned athletes show less cortisol activity after training as their body copes with the stress better. One measure of overtraining is the Testosterone/Cortisol Ratio. Elevated levels of cortisol compared to Testosterone are an indication the athlete is overtraining. If you train with good cycling and rest periods, you are more likely to maintain a constant higher testosterone level whilst keeping cortisol under control. Supplements that actually can increase your testosterone through your testicular axis are vitamin D and Zinc. No other supplements have been proven to significantly do this, so make sure these are adequate in your diet. Another thing to consider, under high cortisol/ or low carbohydrate conditions, gluconeogenesis is derived mainly from Branch Chain Amino Acids (BCAA's) taken from the muscle. These are needed for Glutamine and Alanine synthesis. Extra BCAA's taken during stressful periods, i.e. during or straight after a workout may cause an anticatabolic effect on the muscle, help to initiate protein synthesis and lessen teardown. Recent studies also show the ingestion of Glutamine at this time also prevented the destruction of contractile proteins in muscle.

6) LACK OF SLEEP

Many studies point to sleep being a massive regulator of body function. It helps to maintain vital physiological functions, learning and memory by promoting the regeneration of the central nervous system and cellular recovery. In recent years, a reduction in the duration and quality of sleep in the general population has become evident. This mainly occurs in countries that are heavily industrial and populous. Several studies have been done, highlighting the potential health hazards arising from sleep deprivation. These studies show that poor sleep patterns result in cognitive impairment, poor immune system response, poor metabolism and altered hormonal response. It is generally considered that humans need a good 7-10 hours quality sleep per night. By quality sleep, we mean no more than 3 interruptions of sleep per night.

Sleep deprivation results in 2 distinct outcomes: 1) The increased secretion of Cortisol Hormone, and 2) Changes in the rhythmic secretion of anabolic hormones such as Growth Hormone and Testosterone. Increases in cortisol and decreases in Testosterone can occur after just 24 hours of sleep deprivation. These changes can remain for up to 96 hours. Moreover, further evidence indicates that concentrations of IGF-1 (insulin growth factor 1) secreted by the liver in response to GH (Growth Hormone) are rapidly reduced under periods of sleep deprivation. Considering hormones such as IGF-1, GH and Testosterone are all involved in anabolic protein synthesis, sleep deprivation can have a potentially damaging effect on bodybuilders who wish to improve their gains! IGF-1 mediated signalling is a massive part of signalling protein synthesis in muscle tissue. Testosterone binds to androgen receptors in the cell, telling the cell to upregulate its protein synthesis through transcription of amino acids. Some evidence indicates that testosterone is capable of inhibiting MYOSTATIN. Myostatin is released to inhibit muscle growth by preventing satellite cell r proliferation and differentiation, a critical step in recovery and growth. Elevated levels of cortisol may modulate muscle protein metabolism causing reduced muscle synthesis which further potentiates muscle atrophy. So sleep deprivation damages muscle physiology and impairs muscle recovery because of increased stimulation of protein degradation, so allowing muscles to waste.

CHAPTER 8: WHAT STOPS A MUSCLE RESPONDING
SUMMARY

1) POOR NUTRITION   Make sure that you have good protein sources with all the essential amino acids. Good meat sources are chicken, fish, beef. Other good protein sources are calcium caseinate and whey proteins from milk and cheese (including cottage cheese), eggs. Get approximately 1.6 to 2g protein per kg of bodyweight providing you are less than 15% bodyfat men or 25 % bodyfat women. BCAA's and Glutamine need to be consumed immediately after a workout to prevent too much protein degredation.   Carbohydrate levels should be between 4.8 to 10 g per kg to be protein sparing. Ketogenic diets should be avoided, but at the other end of the scale, only one big insulin spike per day should be achieved by taking simple carbs after a workout and try to just stick to low glycemic carbs the rest of the day. Make sure the post workout drink contains a predigested Hydrolysed whey protein to get the BCAA's into the system quickly.

Make sure you take in essential fatty acids such as fish oils (omega 3's) and omega 6's from nuts and evening primrose oil every day, but don't allow total fat intake to rise above 100g daily.   SCF recommends 6g essential fatty acids for women (5g omega 6, 1g omega 3) and 8g for men (6.4g omega 6, 1.6g omega 3)

MICRONUTRITION   This means we need an adequate supply of vitamins, minerals, trace elements and antioxidants in the diet. Make sure you have adequate supply of vitamins A, D, E and K. These are available from greens, milk, cheese, squash, sweet potato and carrots.
The main antioxidants are Vitamins C and E, selenium and coenzyme Q10. try to get at least 100mg Coenzyme Q10, 200 micrograms selenium, 1000 mg vitamin c and 500IU vitamin E daily.

2 INADEQUATE FLUID INTAKE   Most adult humans need between 2 to 4 litres of water per day depending on bodymass and activity levels. For the strength athlete, this needs to be increased by 40%.

3 OVERTRAINING   Make sure you have adequate rest days and utilise a split system to separate bodyparts. So, try to have one day during the week and 2 days at the weekend resting from heavy resistance training. On a periodisation macrocycle, have a complete week off resistance work every few months.
Use the warm up sets to prepare you for the working set and dont do volume training with supersets, giant sets and the like. Keep time under tension to 1 minute or less. Limit cardio to 2-3 high intensity TABATA sessions weekly, preferably not the same time as your weights workouts. Cycle your training in both planning of exercises, and trying different splits.

4 CONNECTIVE TISSUE STRESS
Cycle your style of training with glycolytic, slow negative and oxidative sessions.

Try to reduce your stress response as much as possible by getting regular soft tissue release treatment sessions and massages. Try to be aware of bad postural positions and deload these regularly by repositioning and stretching. Use core stabilisation techniques to improve internal abdominal activation and postural endurance. Don't for one minute think you have a weak core if you are a bodybuilder, because this isn't correct, just maybe a poor core endurance!

5 HORMONE IMBALANCE The main aim is to reduce the levels of cortisol by adequate carbohydrates and correct proteins in the diet,combined with adequate rest both in between sets and inbetween bodyparts to allow protein synthesis to prevent catabolism taking a hold. To maintain levels of Testosterone and Growth hormones high, adequate Vitamin D and zinc need to be taken.

6 LACK OF SLEEP   Try to get between 7 and 8 hours sleep a night and a power nap of 15 mins during the day

123

Chapter 9
Common Injuries and Conditions Affecting Bodybuilders

We're going to split this chapter up into three headings;

1.   Mechanical Spinal Problems
2.   Tendinopathies, or conditions affecting tendons
3.   Muscular Injuries

1. Mechanical Spinal Problems

Postural Hypertension

As we spoke about in the previous chapter, when we think about the covering over the muscle, i.e. the fascia, when this structure gets tight and restricted, it restricts the circulation to the muscle and, therefore, oxygen supply to the muscle is also restricted. This means other structures, like nerve cells, can also get fatigued, and this shrinkage of the fascia and the inefficient action of the muscles causes postural changes to occur in the body.

As a response of this lack of oxygen to the muscle, the muscle tends to tighten up and the fascia shrinks around it. Depending on which area is affected, this can cause alteration in posture and also dysfunction of other muscle groups through inhibition or an inability to want to contract of the muscle.

If you have a look at the diagram called 'The Stress Response', you can see the chain of events that occurs, and it's almost like a vicious circle.

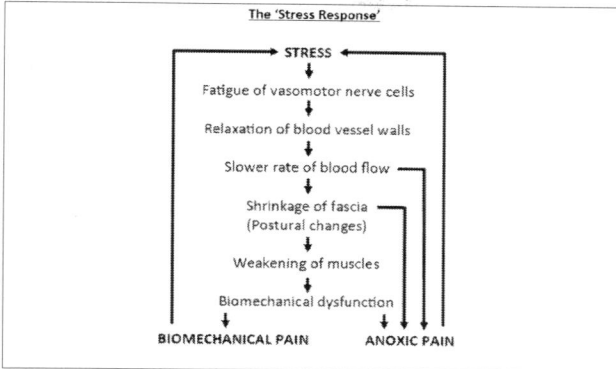

The 'Stress Response'

STRESS

Fatigue of vasomotor nerve cells

Relaxation of blood vessel walls

Slower rate of blood flow

Shrinkage of fascia
(Postural changes)

Weakening of muscles

Biomechanical dysfunction

BIOMECHANICAL PAIN   ANOXIC PAIN

So in other words, when you develop biomechanical pain and anoxic pain, that fuels the stress response and the whole system starts up again. If this cycle continues without any breakage, then the posture becomes hypertensive, and this can lead on to the four types of conditions which we'll now discuss.

A) Facet Joint Syndrome

If we look at the diagram (named 'Facet Joints in Motion') we can see that when we flex forwards and extend backwards there are compressive and traction forces which occur on both the disc and the facet joints where the arrows are pointing.

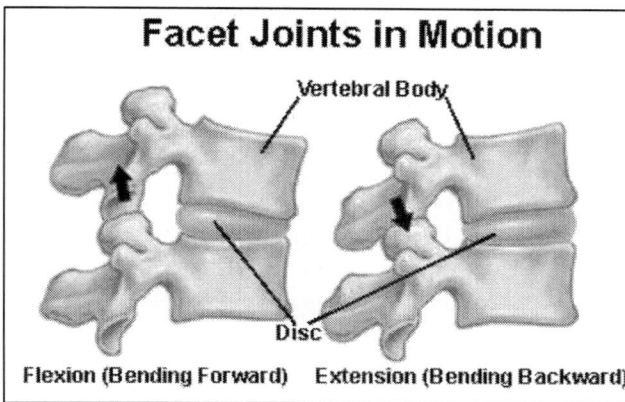

Facet Joints in Motion

Vertebral Body

Disc

Flexion (Bending Forward)   Extension (Bending Backward)

125

In the 1950s there was a famed physician named James Cyriax who postulated the theory that the disc was almost always involved in back pain. Although doctors tend to be brought up with this type of theory, we now know through studies in the type of nerve endings that occur in facet joints and these neural pathways causing pain, that the facet joints are the main causes of pain in acute spinal conditions. Very often, if somebody goes to their GP complaining of pain in the back, they might have some sort of scan or x-ray which shows a degree of degradation in these joints. The doctor will then put this down to a form of osteoarthritis or spondylosis in these joints. Whilst wear of these joints does occur it is important to realise that this situation can be treated. Due to the compressive and torsional forces which occur on the spine in a bodybuilder, we need to be aware that the body will try and adapt to protect these areas. These joints are like any other synovial joint in the body and are protected by ligaments and a capsule.

Through various reflexes that occur, as a protective mechanism, these ligament structures tend to tighten up. This then stiffens these joints and due to the inflammatory debris that is produced can stiffen to such a degree that they adhese together. So the soft tissue structures surrounding these joints can stick and hold the joints in a fixed position. The physiotherapist, when assessing a patient, will firstly look at their posture. Posture tells many a story about what is going on deep down in the facet joints of the spine. If there is a torsional stress and hold on the body, with the surrounding muscles in tension, it's likely that this reflex action (mechanoreceptor reflex) has fired off strongly and is causing a degree of spasm and holding these joints in a tight fashion.

Treatment
The physiotherapist or osteopath will try to alleviate the tension surrounding these joint structures using acupuncture techniques and soft tissue release techniques. This will allow the soft tissues to become more malleable and, therefore, more likely to be released by manipulation techniques. Once these joints are freed off, a series of stretching exercises is given to try and

maintain the freedom in these joints so that this situation of tension is less likely to occur.

Sometimes when patients present with this type of situation the physiotherapist may give core strengthening exercises. This is a bad move because trying to encourage the correct muscles to fire in the right manner when the body wants to shift into an altered posture is very difficult and goes against the grain. The first priority is to free the joints off then improve flexibility and only then should core strengthening and endurance exercises be given.

Thoracic Outlet Syndrome

Very often, bodybuilders tend to over-train with overhead exercises. They might do three or four different pressing movements overhead. This, along with straining when shrugging or deadlifting or squatting, causes tension to build up in the clavicular triangle. This is the notch just behind the clavicle. Thoracic Outlet Syndrome is a disorder that occurs when blood vessels and/or nerves in the space between your collar bone and your first rib are compressed. The artery that runs through this area and the nerves supply blood and nerve signals to all the muscles in the arm. Symptoms can include a decreased pulse and a partial shutdown of blood supply to all the muscles of the arm, resulting in an aching sensation when attempting to use the arm. Sometimes the situation can get so bad that the muscles in the arm can atrophy and performance of bilateral exercises can be very one-sided (see diagram).

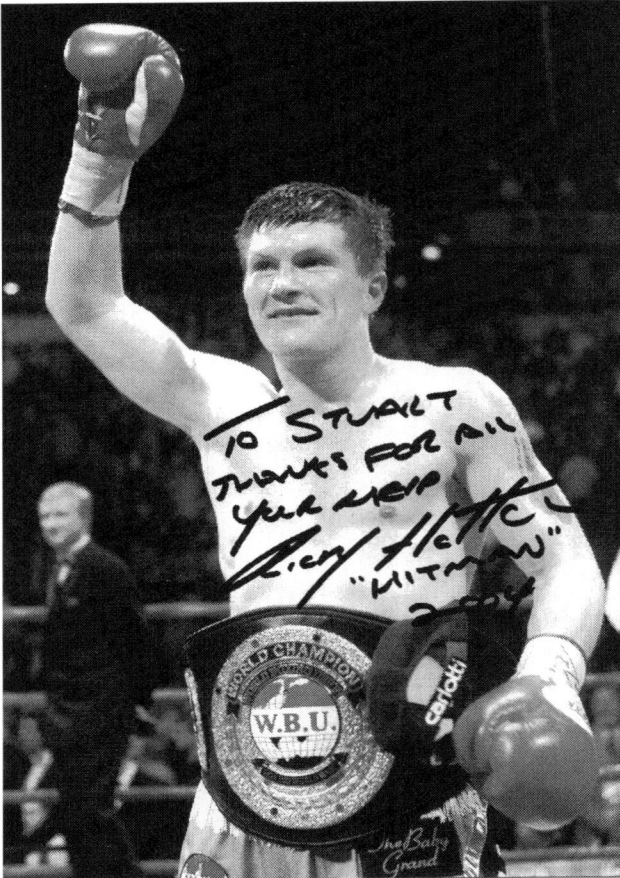

Ricky Hatton: Ricky overcame a number of injuries to become world champion and one of the most successful British boxers ever! I was his Physio for 8 years and Kerry Kayes was his Strength and Nutrition coach.

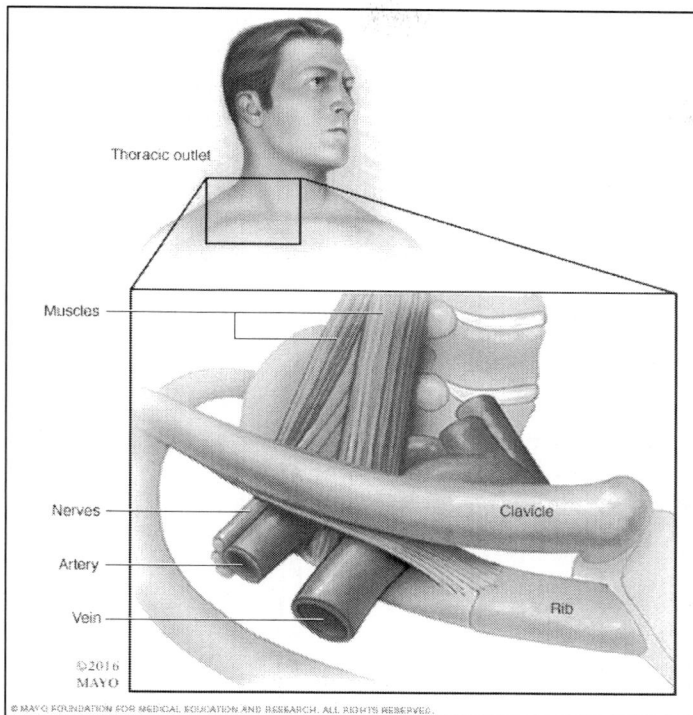

Thoracic outlet

Muscles

Nerves

Clavicle

Artery

Vein

Rib

Treatment

As you can see from the diagram, if the muscles become overused and inflamed, this can cause the soft tissues to adhese to the nerves and the blood vessels. If this is the case, then a combination of acupuncture and manipulation can free these structures off, resulting in an alleviation of pressure on the artery and nerves. This condition is very often misdiagnosed. Some doctors don't even believe it exists. As a physiotherapist for 30 years, in the strength training community, I see this condition many times and it can seriously affect performance.

129

T4 Syndrome

As you may recall, in the previous chapter I mentioned that the automatic control or, if you like, the thermostat regulating the blood flow into both arms is contained from nerve fibres (sympathetic nerve fibres) running on the inside of the rib angles in the upper back. Also in the upper back we have what we call the thoracic vertebrae. So these are the vertebrae that start running from the base of the neck and we can count them T1 to T4.

If these four vertebrae develop tension (similar to Facet Joint Syndrome) then this tension causes muscle spasm in the area. The muscle spasm then decreases the circulatory supply to nerve fibres in the area, which may also include the sympathetic fibres, running along the channels deep to the vertebrae. Small tributary nerves which run off from the sympathetic nerves also run in through the vertebrae. If circulation is altered to these nerves they do not function properly. As a result of that, we get the list of symptoms you can see in the diagram.

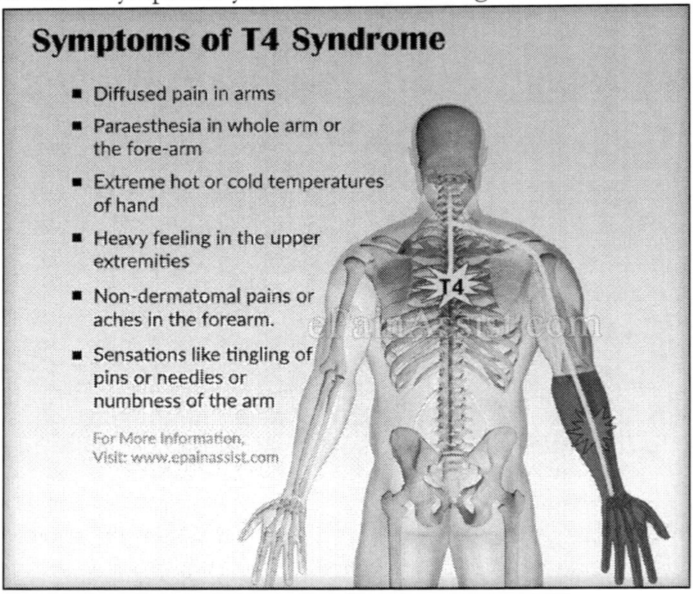

Symptoms of T4 Syndrome

- Diffused pain in arms
- Paraesthesia in whole arm or the fore-arm
- Extreme hot or cold temperatures of hand
- Heavy feeling in the upper extremities
- Non-dermatomal pains or aches in the forearm.
- Sensations like tingling of pins or needles or numbness of the arm

For More Information,
Visit: www.epainassist.com

This can cause a decrease in function in both upper arms and shoulders, and also in the middle back area. Pain can prevent normal function of exercises, especially rowing movement, and also lifting movements using the shoulders. It can include nocturnal pain, and as we all know there's nothing worse than sleep deprivation.

Treatment

Certain acupuncture points are used in two channels running either side of the spine. This allows blood flow to return to these areas. We also use distal acupuncture points running into the arms, to improve the blood flow to the arms. If any joint structures are tight in the thoracic spine these can be released through manipulation techniques and various soft tissue fascial release techniques can be used to improve the malleability of the tissues and, therefore, the blood supply to them. (Some of these techniques can be seen on the DVD)

Tension Headaches (C0/1 Syndrome)

As we see from the diagram called 'Suboccipital Triangle', the back of the head is a very complex area with overlapping muscles and intertwining nerves and blood vessels.

Headache pain can originate from almost anywhere within this complex system. Contraction of the muscles of the head, such as the splenius capitis muscle in the diagram, may stimulate entrapped nerves and cause localised sensation of headache pain to be sent to the brain. This could be as a result of stress or tension, or slight micro tear damage to the muscles due to overexertion or overuse. A network of blood vessels surrounds the head and carries blood to the brain. Abnormal function of this vascular system, sometimes caused by compression of blood vessels by these muscles or tissues in spasm, can also lead to severe headache pain.

The jaw is the most complex joint in the body. It's able to open and close and move side to side and slide forwards and backwards. Muscles and ligaments surrounding the jaw can also

131

be brought into tension and cause compression at the side of the head resulting in temporal or side headache pain. Disorders of the neck muscles or the bones of the cervical spine may also cause pain in this area where the disorder occurs and transmit pain to an area at the back of the head where it's experienced as a headache. Lower down the shoulder and back muscles can also be affected by tension which can then transmit to muscles higher up, especially the trapezius muscle which, again, attaches to the base of the skull and can cause compression to these nerves and blood vessels in this area.

Suboccipital Triangle

Rectus capitis posterior minor muscle
Rectus capitis posterior major muscle
Epicranial aponeurosis (galea aponeurotica)
Occipital belly (occipitalis) of occipitofrontalis muscle
Semispinalis capitis muscle (cut and reflected)
Greater occipital nerve (dorsal ramus of C2 spinal nerve)
Vertebral artery (atlantic part)
Occipital artery
Obliquus capitis superior muscle
Suboccipital nerve (dorsal ramus of C1 spinal nerve)
3rd (least) occipital nerve (dorsal ramus of C3 spinal nerve)
Posterior arch of atlas (C1 vertebra)
Occipital artery
Semispinalis capitis muscle in posterior triangle of neck
Obliquus capitis inferior muscle
Splenius capitis muscle in posterior triangle of neck
Greater occipital nerve (dorsal ramus of C2 spinal nerve)
Posterior auricular artery
Splenius capitis muscle (cut and reflected)
Great auricular nerve (cervical plexus C2, 3)
3rd (least) occipital nerve (dorsal ramus of C3 spinal nerve)
Longissimus capitis muscle
Lesser occipital nerve (cervical plexus C2, 3)
Splenius cervicis muscle
Sternocleidomastoid muscle
Semispinalis cervicis muscle
Trapezius muscle
Semispinalis capitis muscle (cut)
Posterior cutaneous branches of dorsal rami of C4, 5, 6 spinal nerves
Splenius capitis muscle (cut)

Causes of Tension Headaches
- Dehydration
- Tiredness
- Change of Activities
- Postural Tension
- Lack of Activity
- Poor Mobility

132

People often ask, "What is the difference between a migraine and a tension headache?" Below, there are two lists of symptoms to differentiate between the two.

MIGRAINES	TENSION HEADACHES
Visual disturbances, strange lights, prisms.	No visual phenomena, just difficult to focus and concentrate.
Light and noise can play a role.	Light and noise make little difference to symptoms.
Pain usually affects one side of the head but can be associated with nausea and vomiting.	It can affect the whole head (the frontal and the temporal areas). It doesn't usually cause nausea.
Exercise can trigger a migraine.	Exercise in general can relieve the tension through increased blood flow. However, over-exercising and creating more tension in the extensor muscles of the neck can increase the symptoms.

Treatment
The first main aim is to release the tension in the muscles down the back of the head, and the back and the side of the neck. Acupuncture technique works well for this, sometimes with additional electro-stimulation. Once a degree of tension is released in the soft tissues, then any hard tissues can be manipulated and freed off. As a result of strong tension at the base of the skull, the area called C0/1 gets very tightly clamped together. This is the articulation between the top of the neck and the base of the skull. This facet joint is very large and is held strongly by ligamentous structures. If the muscles

surrounding this joint clamp the joint together too strongly it can literally stick. This, in turn, causes a strong reflex (mechanoreceptor reflex) to initiate even stronger contraction of the surrounding muscles. So this is a self-replicating condition. This also increases the tension headache to such a degree where the pain can be excruciating.

We do a special manipulation on this joint by getting the head in a certain position, as seen on the DVD, to literally release the tension in this facet joint. This can then alleviate or negate the need for this reflex action resulting in muscle relaxation and improved blood flow.

2. Tendinopathies (Damage to tendons)

A) Rotator Cuff Problems

If we look at the diagram named 'Rotator Cuff Tear' we can see that your shoulder joint is a ball and socket joint held in position by a cuff of four muscles that come together as tendons to form a covering around the head of the humerus.

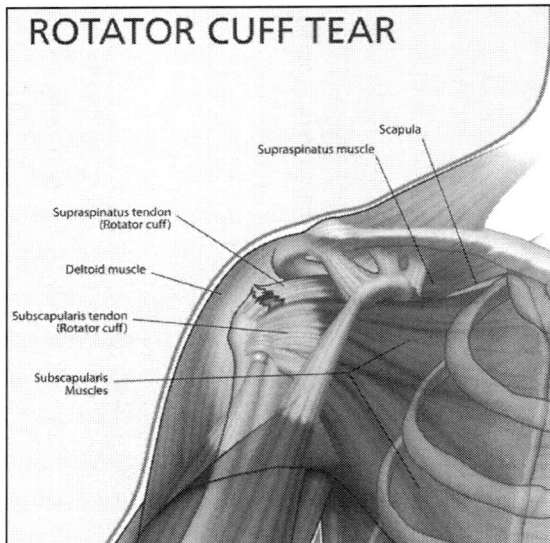

ROTATOR CUFF TEAR

Scapula
Supraspinatus muscle
Supraspinatus tendon (Rotator cuff)
Deltoid muscle
Subscapularis tendon (Rotator cuff)
Subscapularis Muscles

The rotator cuff attaches the humerus to the shoulder blade and it helps to lift and rotate your arm. These muscles work together to stabilise the ball in a shallow socket. Without these muscles working together, the shoulder would be completely unstable. The four muscles are called supraspinatus, subscapularis and on the back of the shoulder infraspinatus and teres minor. As you can see on the diagram, the tendon that is torn is called supraspinatus. This is probably the most common tendon to be torn with bodybuilders. Under normal circumstances, this tendon is torn acutely when you fall down on an outstretched arm or lift something too heavy with a jerking motion. Although this can be the situation with bodybuilders, maybe doing a snatching movement, usually the movement should be more controlled and this is unlikely to be the case.

The type of tear that occurs with bodybuilders is called a degenerative tear. These are the result of a wearing down of the tendon that occurs slowly over time. This degeneration can occur naturally as we age but in bodybuilding circles it's usually either due to overtraining or training with poor form, where a repetitive stress is placed on the tendon. Very often with bodybuilders, there tends to be a predisposition to overuse of the anterior shoulder structures, including a muscle called pectoralis minor and subscapularis. These develop undue tension causing the anterior shoulder capsule to tighten and the shoulder is held in a forward protracted position. This can cause more friction to occur on the supraspinatus tendon and when a person does heavy pressing movements this can increase the repetitive stress on the tendon. Overuse and overtraining don't allow the tendon time to recover. Therefore, micro tears can build up and eventually lead to a larger tear. As the posture of the shoulder alters and becomes asymmetrical, this can also affect the blood supply to the tendon because as structures get tighter it limits the blood supply and, therefore, the ability of the body to repair tendon damage is impaired. Another factor is, due to stress on these structures, bone spurs can occur on the underside of the acromion bone in the shoulder, and this can impinge on the tendon and can weaken it over time and make it more likely to tear.

Symptoms

Very often there is pain at rest and also at night, particularly if lying on the affected shoulder. There is also pain when lifting the arm out to the side and lowering the arm slowly. When lifting or rotating the arm there is a degree of weakness in this area. Also, crepitus or a crackling sensation can occur when moving your shoulder in certain positions.

Treatment

Depending on the degree of tear, if it is a full thickness tear, i.e. through the full thickness of the tendon, usually surgery is the only option here. If there is only a partial thickness tear, then physiotherapy, as demonstrated on the DVD, and also a technique called PRP injections (Platelet Rich Plasma) where growth factors from the platelets in your own blood can improve the repair of the tendon. With regard to physiotherapy, very often alongside direct treatment of this rotator cuff tear, such as ultrasound, laser and localised soft tissue techniques, we can also analyse the posture of the shoulder including the scapula (shoulder blade). As demonstrated on the video, very often the shoulder blade can dysfunction. When the shoulder is in a protracted or forward placed position, it can often lead to an inhibition of muscles on the back of the shoulder controlling the scapula position. This further leads to postural dysfunction of the shoulder leading to inhibition of muscular contractions and also can lead to more degeneration in the shoulder tendons. By applying certain exercises to these shoulder blade muscles, we can control and improve shoulder posture to alleviate these problems in the future.

B) Epicondylitis

The most common name for this type of condition is golfer's elbow or tennis elbow. This is a degeneration of the common flexor tendon on the inside of the elbow or the common extensor tendon on the outside of the elbow. It is usually caused not by a direct trauma but by repetitive strain over time.

In bodybuilding, due to the repetitive nature of movements such as cleaning and curling this puts an undue stress repeatedly on the attachment of the muscles on the back of the forearm or the inside of the forearm. As you can see on the diagram, there are a number of muscles which all work together, which attach to the outside of the elbow and this is the area which is generally affected.

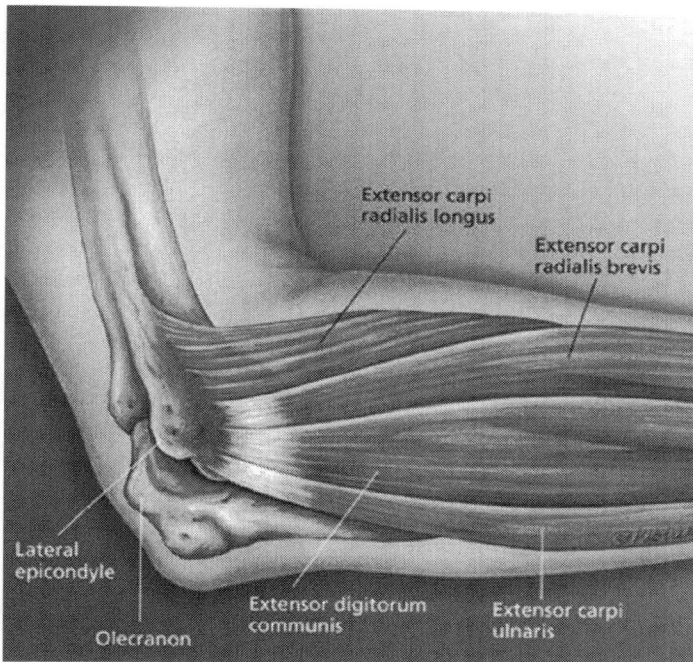

Symptoms

These include pain on the outside or the inside of the elbow, varying from sharp to intense dull aching. Sharp pain usually occurs when attempting to grip something and lift it off upwards. For example, lifting a kettle or an iron. Nocturnal pain can be a dull ache intermittently and also a tender area locally on the bone, on the outside or the inside of the elbow. Very often with bodybuilders, there will be dull initial signs that may be ignored and as training continues, the symptoms may worsen.

137

Treatment
Localised physiotherapy techniques such as ultrasound, laser and acupuncture needling can be used to improve circulatory supply to these tendons to help them repair quicker. With the latest research into tendinopathies it is now commonly agreed that a tendon needs to be loaded to a certain degree to allow it to heal properly. As physiotherapists, we are careful to continually reassess the loading capability of the tendon, being careful not to overload but apply enough loading to effect healing. One of the best ways of doing this is using eccentric work or slow negative contractions, for instance the lowering of a weight slowly from wrist extended position to wrist flexion, lifting a small weight in this manner. Isometric contractions at different ranges can also be employed to assist the healing of the tendon. It has been demonstrated that eccentric work increases MGF (Mechano Growth Factors) and also stimulates collagen realignment and production.

C) Anterior Knee Pain

Anterior knee pain is pain that occurs at the front and centre of the knee. It can be caused by many different problems, including; chondromalacia of the patella, which is a softening and breakdown of the cartilage on the underside of the kneecap; patella mal-tracking, which is an instability of the patella on the knee; quadriceps tendinitis, which is a pain and tenderness of the quadriceps tendon attaching to the patella, either underneath or on top. These conditions can be interlinked and there is usually a mechanical or an overuse reason for them.

Causes
If you look at the diagram 'Tendons of the Knee' you'll notice that your kneecap (patella) sits over the front of your knee joint.

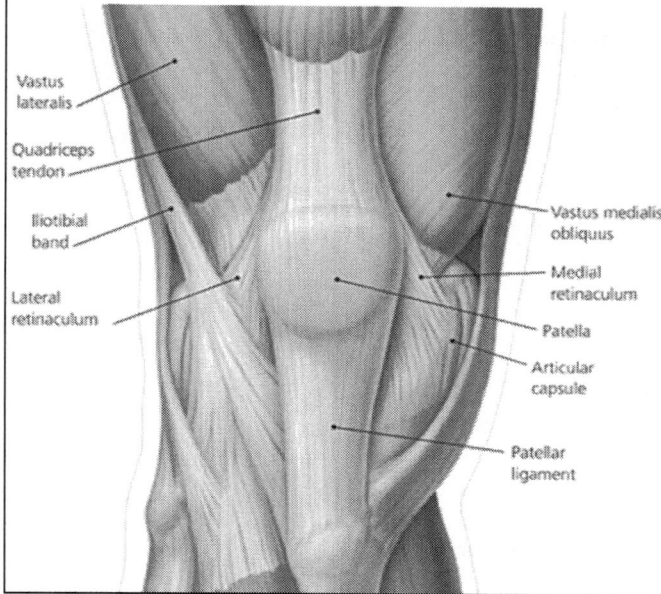

Tendons of the Knee

Vastus lateralis

Quadriceps tendon

Iliotibial band

Lateral retinaculum

Vastus medialis obliquus

Medial retinaculum

Patella

Articular capsule

Patellar ligament

As you bend or straighten your knee, the underside of the patella glides over the bones that make up the knee. Strong tendons help attach the kneecap to the bones and muscles that surround the knee. These tendons are called the patella tendons which attach the kneecap to the shin bone, and the quadriceps tendon, which attaches the kneecap to the quadriceps muscle. Anterior knee pain usually begins when the kneecap doesn't move properly and rubs against the lower part of the thigh bone. This may occur because the kneecap is in an abnormal position, a poor alignment, which could be caused through tightness or weakness of muscles on the front and the back of the thigh and also the sides of the attachment to the patella. When looking at mechanical causes one also has to look at the joints that occur above and below the knee. So we look at the hip, including gluteal muscles that may be tight or tight rotators of the hip. We also look at the tibia, which is the shin bone, whether or not there is some tibial torsion occurring which also could be due to a person having flat feet or a rotational element at the ankle or the heel.

Once we analyse all these postural effects, we can correct these by either exercise or orthotics for the feet, and this will allow the knee to be more in alignment. When we look at the patella itself, we can apply certain treatment modalities to try and release tension from around the sides of the kneecap and then also administer exercises to try and allow certain muscle groups to balance so the kneecap glides smoothly. With regard to overuse of the knee tendons, i.e. the patella tendon and the quadriceps tendon, we can employ slow negative or eccentric work, usually in a squatting position or in a position where the quadriceps has to work to apply a loading to the tendon to allow it to heal quicker. Localised physiotherapy techniques such as laser and ultrasound can be applied to speed the healing process.

D) Traction Apophysitis Triceps

This is almost a unique condition which bodybuilders can get. It involves overuse of the tricep attachment to the olecranon, the point of the elbow. The triceps is utilised in any kind of pressing movement and then obviously strongly utilised when performing extension movements. There is a lot of tension on this tendon, especially when performing extension movements of the elbow in an overhead position. Jerky technique along with a tendency to over train without adequate rest leads to a micro tear build up and sometimes bony spur build up on the point of the olecranon, hence the term traction apophysitis. This can get inflamed and the tendon can also degrade right on the point of attachment. Occasionally, this can lead to rupture but usually it's characterised by a partial degrading of the tendon as a result of overuse. Symptoms include pain when the elbow is extended from a fully flexed position, even with a light weight, pain when resting on the elbow. Treatment is the same as is applied to other tendinopathies.

3. Muscular Injuries

Although bodybuilders may tear any muscle that is trained, the most common muscular injuries to occur with bodybuilders are pectoral tears and muscle slides, and compression type syndromes such as the one that occurs commonly at the brachialis and brachioradialis intersection, at the elbows.

A) Pectoral Tears/Muscle Slides

If we look at the two diagrams, on the first diagram we see there is the attachment of the pectoral muscle to the humerus.

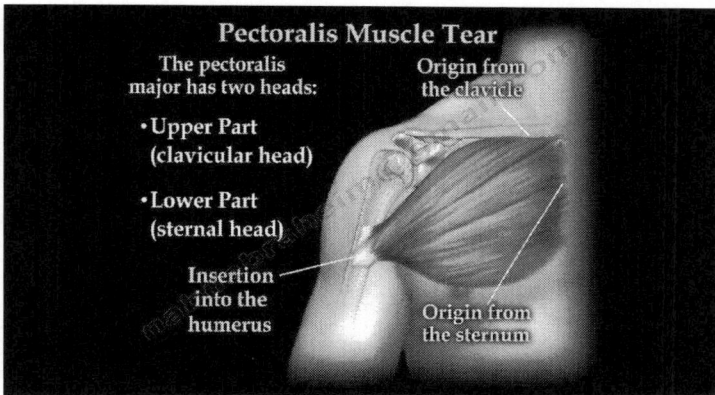

Pectoralis Muscle Tear

The pectoralis major has two heads:

• Upper Part (clavicular head)

• Lower Part (sternal head)

Origin from the clavicle

Insertion into the humerus

Origin from the sternum

This is a broad attachment and there are three parts to the pectoral. Although the diagram shows the upper part and the lower part, there is a midsection. The pectoral is called the multipennate muscle, which means that the fibres come in at different angles. So the clavicular portion comes in from an upper angle and the sternal head, lower part of the pectoral, comes in from a lower angle. Tears in this muscle most commonly occur during the bench press. The bench press is a nonspecific compound pressing movement which involves the anterior deltoid, the pectoral and the tricep muscles. As these three muscle groups are involved, if there is a weakness in any one it can overstress another.

141

In my experience, one of the most common reasons for tears in the pectoral is a combination of the following;

1. The fact that most bodybuilders tend to use compound pressing movements far too often in their training regimes.

2. The bench press, which is really a nonspecific compound exercise, is over-utilised and not necessary for bodybuilding training.

3. Bodybuilders that use anabolic steroids have sudden leaps in strength increases. The muscle recovers quickly from these, but the tendon has a much slower metabolism and recovers much slower. As the bodybuilder tends to over-press, the muscle tendon junction gets put under stress and can give way. This causes a muscle slide as you can see in the picture which shows an indentation in the pectoral muscle.

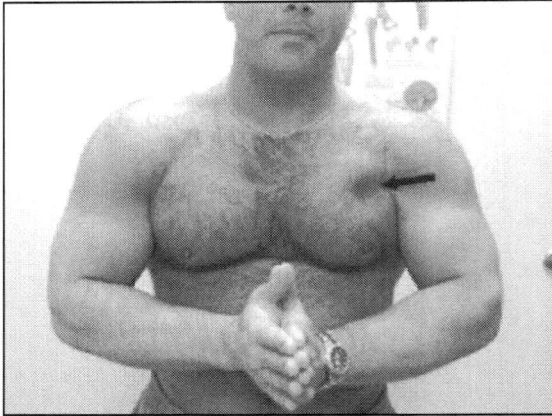

In this situation, the tendon hasn't torn off the bone, but the muscle has slid from its junction with the tendon and caused a large tear in the area. Symptoms include sudden sharp pain in this area, profuse bleeding down the arm and the side of the body, temporary loss in function or weakness in the pectoral.

Treatment involves removal of the exudate or the protein debris from this inflammatory reaction, electrotherapy techniques such as laser and ultrasound to improve the healing of the muscle tendon junction, and then this is followed by slow graduated eccentric work at different angles to involve the pectoral muscle tendon junction and to speed the healing process.

B) Compressive and Micro tear Injuries

The other type of muscular injury we deal with for bodybuilders is the compressive and micro tear type injuries such as the one that occurs at the elbow, usually involving the brachialis and brachioradialis muscles. As you can see from the diagram, the brachioradialis muscle is quite a long muscle attaching over the elbow, and it is a long flexor of the elbow, especially when your forearm is pronated or in the mid position.

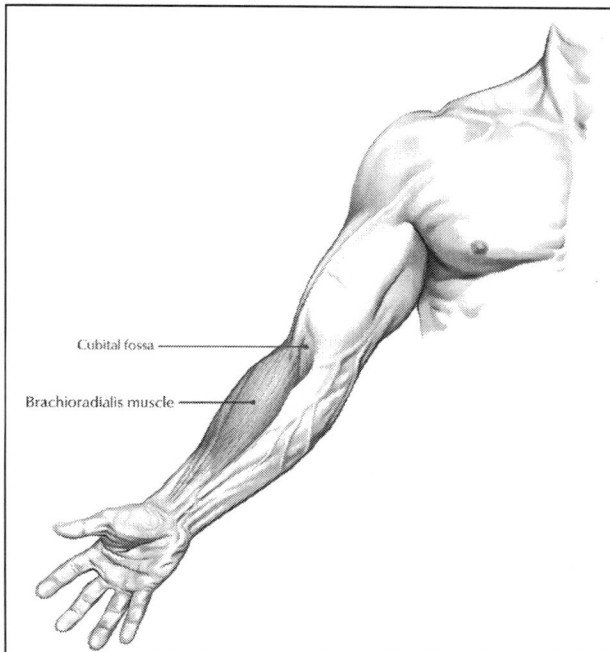

Cubital fossa

Brachioradialis muscle

Additionally, it supports the extension of the wrist. It is used very often in flexion movements in bodybuilding. As it's a long flexor shunt muscle and not a spurt muscle like the biceps, it gets prone to overuse near the elbow area, especially when performing cleaning movements with a sudden sharp flick of the wrist as well. This can form micro tears which build up at the top end of the muscle causing inflammation and swelling which, in turn, can compress nerve and blood vessel structures deep under the belly of the muscle. If this situation persists, the compressive forces increase, it can also involve the brachialis muscle which is deep to it in the cubital fossa area of the elbow, as seen on the diagram. Typical pain response from this injury is a dull ache and sometimes an inability to grip the bar, a feeling of wanting to release your grip because of the pain at the top end of the elbow. It can become so bad that you find it difficult to pick up a glass or a cup. Treatment usually starts by advising how to train around this area and avoid overtraining this muscle. Once the new training regime is underway as well, treatment involves localised treatment to heal the tissues, deep kneading and superficial fascial release techniques and trigger point acupuncture locally helps to improve circulation and release pressure.

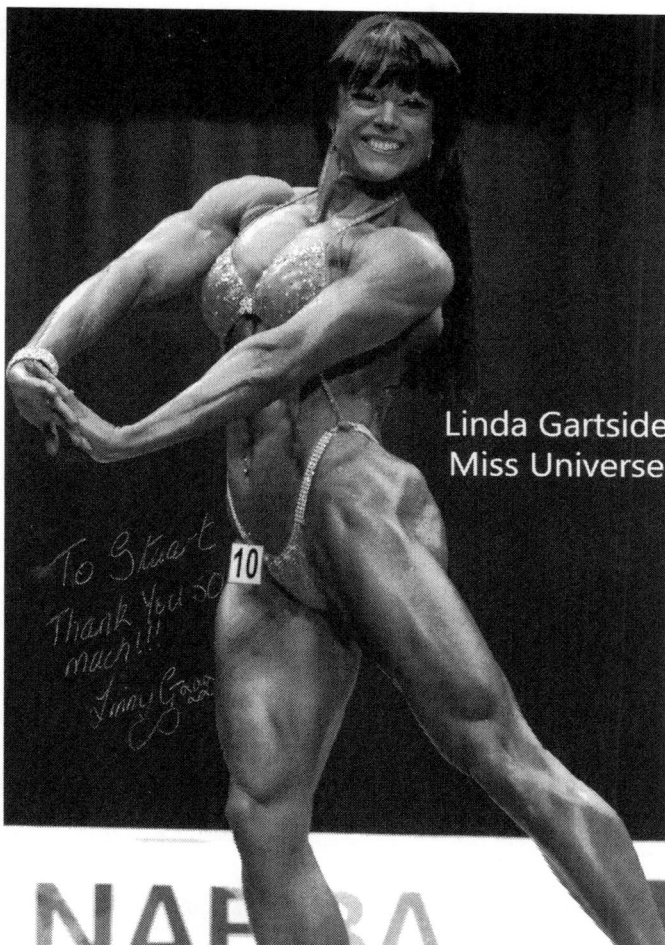

Linda Gartside
Miss Universe

To Stuart
Thank You so
much!!!
Linda Gartside

Linda Gartside: Through courage and determination, Linda now has a Universe Title and is now Professional. I am proud to have helped her through some debilitating injuries!

Chapter 9 – Common Injuries & Conditions Affecting Bodybuilders – Summary

1. Mechanical Spinal Problems

When muscles tighten through overuse or poor posture, the fascia, connective tissue that surrounds the muscle, tightens. As this tightens, it restricts the circulation coming in and out of the muscle and it's also highly sensitive. There are a lot of sensory nerve endings in this structure so this gives rise to pain as it becomes more tight. If we have another look at the picture of 'The Stress Response', as you can see this can be a repeated cycle of events.

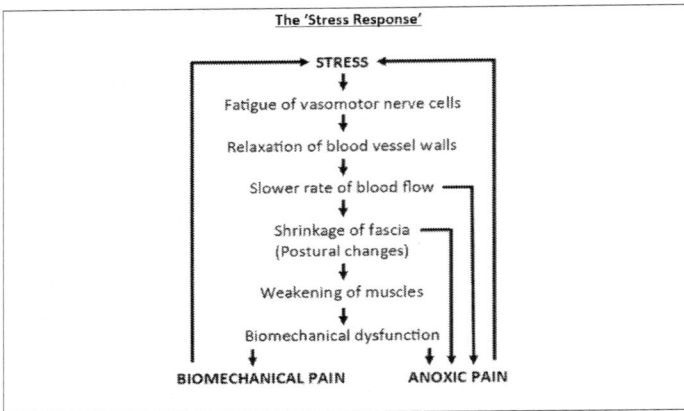

```
                    The 'Stress Response'

                    ──► STRESS ◄──
                           ↓
           Fatigue of vasomotor nerve cells
                           ↓
            Relaxation of blood vessel walls
                           ↓
              Slower rate of blood flow ───
                           ↓
                 Shrinkage of fascia ───
                 (Postural changes)
                           ↓
               Weakening of muscles
                           ↓
             Biomechanical dysfunction
                           ↓
    BIOMECHANICAL PAIN          ANOXIC PAIN
```

It can lead to further tension and further loss of blood flow and oxygen to the muscle tissues. The posture can change so much that muscles can be inhibited to contract. If this is the case, very often performance levels drop in the gym. Intervention is required at this stage, otherwise the situation could get really chronic, making it harder to rectify the problem in the future. All four of these syndromes listed here may be brought on by this type of situation.

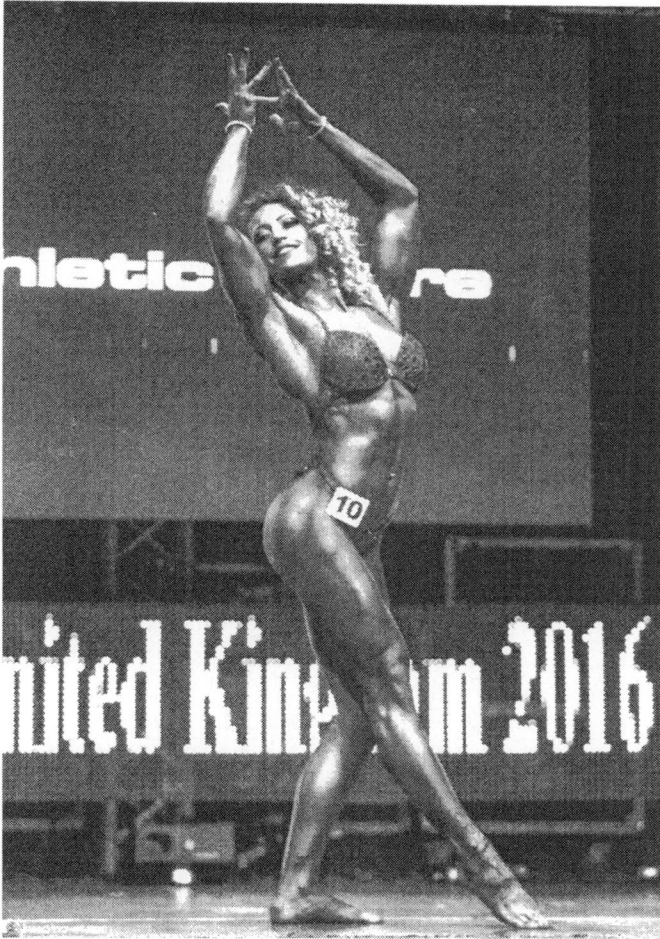

Charlotte MacGill: Charlotte was practically anorexic when she came to me as a student. I managed to inculcate into her the benefits of this style of training and nutrition and here is the end result!! Charlotte won Miss Universe in the Toned figure class with this amazing shape! She also acquired numerous other National and International titles. She now works for me as one of our physios!

Facet Joint Syndrome

This tends to affect the lower facet joints of the spine and can be brought about, as we said before, through this postural hypertension or it could be brought on by severe trauma.

Thoracic Outlet Syndrome

This tends to affect an artery and a nerve system coming from the base of the neck supplying the arms. Any tension in this area can lead to symptoms of altered sensation and circulation into the arms.

T4 Syndrome

This affects the upper area of the back and can also affect the circulation supply to the arms.

Tension Headaches (C0/1 Syndrome)

These can be brought about by extreme tension in the extensors or the neck muscles at the back clamping the skull to the neck. This can be brought on by poor posture, anxiety or stress and also repeated trauma of the muscles at the back of the neck, usually through poor training technique.

Treatment for all these syndromes is by acupuncture, manipulation and mobilisation techniques. Their main effect is to improve the blood flow to the structures and also to relax the muscles. Postural re-education follows on from this where the patient is given a series of postural rehabilitation exercises to help to maintain their good posture.

2. Tendinopathies (Damaged Tendons)

A) Rotator Cuff Problems

Rotator cuff injuries can be brought about either by direct trauma or a combination of poor posture and repeated trauma causing a degradation of the tendons involved in the rotator cuff. Either prior to this injury or as a direct result of this injury, scapula dysfunction may result. This can make the situation worse causing more pressure on the tendons and can also inhibit some of the prime mover muscles required to perform overhead movements especially. Where there is inhibition of the muscles on the back of the scapula less control occurs in the main shoulder joint leading to further shoulder problems. Treatment of these injuries is a direct treatment to the tendons using acupuncture, ultrasound and soft tissue techniques, followed by a re-education of the scapula posture and also the glenohumeral posture of the main shoulder joint. This is by means of re-education exercises given that the patient can do in the gym as warm up prior to doing shoulder movements. Advice is given regarding shoulder movements to avoid overhead movements initially and to maintain a good control of the stabilising muscles during the exercise.

Subheadings B) Epicondylitis, C) Anterior Knee Pain and D) Traction Apophysitis are all linked to either repetitive stress or overuse injuries. Very often with bodybuilding a lot of time is allowed for the muscle to recover but not enough time for the tendons, and as a result of that, tendons tend to get overused and can degrade. The collagen fibres can be damaged and not allowed to recover in time. Changes in the tissue over time can cause them to degrade and become more painful and inefficient. Treatment involves modifying the exercises in bodybuilding to be less ballistic and explosive. More controlled eccentric work is utilised to help to retrain the tendons and to recover the collagen fibres. This can act as a double whammy, helping the muscle to regain size and strength as we know that it can do very easily with eccentric exercise. Modification of some of the exercises is also done, either restricting the range, which is painful, or slightly altering the angles involved.

3. Muscular Injuries

As the muscles in bodybuilders can get strong very quickly, especially when utilising ergogenic aids, as we now know the metabolism in the muscle is much faster than that of the tendon due to the slow turnover of the tendon and the fast turnover of the muscle, the muscle tendon junction becomes at risk. Most of the injuries occur at this junction due to massive gains in strength without periodising your routine.

It was once thought anabolic steroids were directly responsible for injuries such as pec tears, but we know now that this isn't the case. Anabolic steroids are, as the name suggests, anabolic and not catabolic with regard to tendon and muscle tendon junction structures. In my experience this is primarily due to overzealous bodybuilding in the early stages without factoring in eccentric work. To be honest, there aren't too many top professional bodybuilders performing eccentric work like we used to have in the 70s.

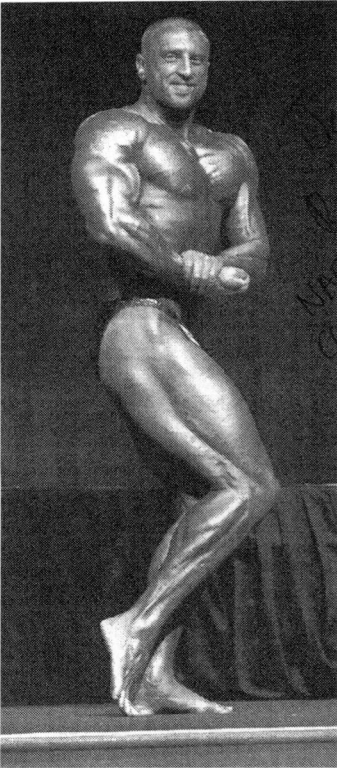

John Ramsay: John came to work for me after finishing his Physio degree. He applied these training principles and achieved this condition coming close to winning the prestigious North west Championships. He too is part of Team Cosgrove and is now engaged to be married to Charlotte!!

Chapter 10 – Off Season and Pre Contest Nutrition Plans

1. Off-Season Diet

Before we start, it would be good to look at some common mistakes that are made during off-season dieting.

a) Not working out your metabolism. Before embarking on a diet, it is useful to know how many calories you need to take in to at least sustain your body weight, or if wishing to gain or lose how many extra calories are needed to take in maybe on a cyclical basis. In order to do this it would be wise to work out how many calories you take in over a seven day period. Once you've made a note of everything you eat and drink over this seven day period, making a diary daily, then you total your calories and then divide by seven to find out your average daily intake. Provided your body weight hasn't changed during that seven days, you could assume that you have burnt off all those calories in the week. This would give you your effective Basal Metabolic Rate, or BMR during normal activities. Any sudden, sharp increases in your body weight would have to be assumed to be fat or water. Each pound of fat would amount to an excess of 3,500 calories, so this would have to be allowed for.

b) Not cycling carbohydrates enough, resulting in fat accumulation or decreased muscle gains.

c) Bulking up, i.e. ingesting too many calories over a long period of time, resulting in an accumulation of fat.

d) Ingesting too much of the wrong type of fat.

e) Not eating enough greens and fibre.

151

f)   Not eating the right type of protein at the right time and either taking too little or too much protein.

2. Macros

Protein
When we look at protein requirements in intensely trained strength athletes such as bodybuilders, it's generally accepted now that the studies done by Dr Michael Colgan back in the 80s are also substantiated by more modern research culminating in guidelines set up in 2009 by the nutrition and athletic performance paper from the American College of Sports Medicine. It tends to agree that this requirement is 1.4 to 1.7 grams per kilogram of bodyweight. Now, this is providing the athlete is relatively lean even in the off season. We're looking at body fat percentages of no more than 15 percent here. If you're working in pounds, this would result in a 200lb strength athlete requiring a protein intake of at least 200 grams per day. If we split this 200 gram daily requirement up into six equal portions, it would result in an intake per meal of 33 to 35 grams per portion. This happens to be the optimum dose that studies suggest needs to be taken in per meal to maximise muscle protein synthesis. Anything substantially more than this ingestion would result in the protein being oxidised for energy rather than utilised to synthesize new tissue. The way round this kind of ingestion of protein is making sure that the protein isn't always taken just on its own. If we add in the fats and carbohydrates, ingesting a mixed meal, this then can improve the uptake of the protein due to slowing down the digestive process and the amino acid delivery to the muscle cells. This would mean that maybe up to 70 grams of protein could be taken at any one time if the protein was combined with carbohydrates and fats which would decrease the rate of protein breakdown and, therefore, increase the protein used for protein synthesis of new tissue. It's possible then that you could increase the daily intake up to 2.3 to 2.5 grams per kilogram, or up to 1.5 grams per pound of bodyweight. This would act as an insurance even if some of the amino acids were oxidised for energy. When cellular uptake of amino acids is relatively slower during the day, then it's a good idea to take in combined meals and also to take

152

in a protein which is combined, i.e. more than one source, so that a slow, steady influx of amino acids is available. An example of this would be to take in a milk based protein rather than just a pure whey protein during the day. When we look at protein powders for supplementation, during the day we would look for something with micellar casein in which gets converted to a bolus in the stomach and is broken down slowly over a period of six to seven hours. This would be less likely to oxidise as energy and be more used for protein synthesis, whereas post workout we would be looking at something like a whey based protein, especially a whey protein isolate, such as hydrolysed whey. This is a partially pre-digested whey which is available within the first 30 minutes following a workout.

Post workout, when the catabolic process of tearing the muscle down begins, a group of amino acids called branched chain amino acids are lost from the muscle. Also lost is an amino acid called glutamine which stands out as by far the most potent amino acid to counteract the catabolic process and to rehydrate the cell. It is necessary to replace both these groups of amino acids, the branched chains and the glutamine. This begins the process of counteracting catabolism and beginning the anabolic process to re-establish the protein matrix. Within two hours after exercise, the glutamine infusion also increases muscle glycogen more than any other amino acid. So, providing the carbohydrates are present, as in the form of sugars, post workout, this response occurs. When we look at other protein sources, we also need to make sure that we have a good balance to make sure that we have a good amino acid profile, ensuring all the essential amino acids are present. For example, eggs contain the sulphurous amino acids which other proteins don't always have. Also, red meat contains iron and creatine to replenish the muscle supplies. White fish has a very low fat and high protein ratio. I would suggest that, of the protein sources taken in per day, two should be from protein drinks, one post workout drink, and the rest from a mixture of dietary proteins such as fish, red meat, chicken and eggs.

Fats

When we look at the current dietary guidelines for strength athletes, they tend to recommend 20 to 30 percent of the total calories taken in per day should come from fats. They also recommend that of that intake ten percent of the fat should come from monounsaturated sources, and ten percent polyunsaturated sources, and less than 10 percent from saturated fats or animal fats. Now, let's try and simplify that a bit more and be more beneficial to the athlete.

When we think about fats, we think about fats breaking down to fatty acids which are required by the body. Providing the body gets two groups of fats, Omega-6s and Omega-3s, it can then manufacture the required fatty acids to maintain health and metabolism and also muscle growth. Fats are also responsible for hormone production so it's necessary that you get the right type of fatty acids in your diet. A lot of research has been done, especially recently, stating the fact that the ratio of Omega-6s to Omega-3s is ridiculously high in the general population. By studying the average American diet, it's been proven that the ratio of Omega-6 to Omega-3 is ten-to-one (10:1). The downside of this is that some unhealthy side effects occur, including increased chance of cardiovascular problems, increased inflammatory response and decrease of hormones such as testosterone. The good news is we can improve this ratio of Omega-6 to Omega-3s quite drastically simply by reducing our percentage intake of fat calories from 20 down to 10. We've got to be careful that we don't lower our dietary intake below ten percent as that can affect hormone response and can prove to be unhealthy. So if we don't drop below ten, we improve our ratio, but also if we think about the content of our fats, if we get healthy fats such as nuts, if we think of changing our intake of nuts from almonds to walnuts, that increases our Omega-3s and decreases our Omega-6s. Similarly, cooking oils such as sunflower oil high in Omega-6s, if we switch to flax seed oil this improves our ratio. If we also increase our intake of oily fish such as salmon and mackerel, this also increases our Omega-3s and reduces our ratio down to two-to-one (2:1), or three-to-one (3:1).

154

Overall, in conclusion, our fat intake should be from the following sources:

• Nuts (in the right balance)
• Oils, such as flax seed oil
• Oily fish, such as salmon and mackerel
• Coconut oil, which has health benefits and contains medium chain fatty acids.
• Keep our animal fat sources down to a minimum

Carbohydrates

It's important that athletes take enough carbohydrates to provide energy for intense resistance exercise. It's important that blood sugar levels are maintained within normal limits to fuel this exercise. Carbohydrates are also necessary to replenish glycogen stores which are also used to fuel the necessary protein synthesis to rejuvenate the muscle tissue. Although the recommended daily carbohydrate intake for intense athletes ranges from six to ten grams per kilogram bodyweight, this can vary depending on the athlete's requirements. During the rest of the day it's important that carbohydrates should be more complex in nature and also from low Glycemic Index type of carbohydrate, i.e. one that doesn't suddenly fluctuate blood sugar levels when taken in. Sources available are:

• Basmati rice
• Pasta
• Granular or whole grain bread products
• Fruits
• Sweet potatoes
• Potatoes
• Fibrous carbohydrates from various vegetables

It's interesting to note that whilst during the day blood sugar levels need to be kept within reasonable levels, straight after a workout it's very important to ingest simple sugars which go straight into the system to cause a sharp insulin response. It's a catch 22 with insulin, because insulin is one of the most powerful anabolic hormones available which immediately

155

improves muscle glycogen and amino acid uptake causing a massive protein synthesis response, and yet it also allows a higher storage of fat than normal. So providing the insulin response is only once daily, straight after a workout there will be no fat storage from this and just maximises the anabolic response.

Pre and Post Workout Drinks

With regard to pre workout drinks, the main aim of a pre workout drink is to hydrate and stimulate. By stimulate we mean to mainly improve the energy response or energy production during the workout. In the first line of defence with regard to resistance exercise, the initial energy response comes from creatine. So it would make sense to supplement your pre workout drink with creatine. Creatine is amongst the most well-researched and effective supplements out there. It could help with exercise performance by rapidly producing energy during intense activity. Creatine is a molecule produced in the body and it stores high energy phosphate groups in the form of phosphocreatine. This releases energy to aid cellular function during stress. This effect causes strength increases after creatine supplementation. Although it's found in some foods, mostly meat, eggs and fish, supplementation can make sure that you have the necessary amount available to get you through the workout. Whenever you take creatine, make sure you take enough water with it because if you don't it can cause stomach cramping and diarrhoea. Don't try to take too much at once, the dose can be spread out during the day as well as in the pre workout drink. Don't take any more than five grams in any one sitting, and contrary to popular belief it's not necessary to load this supplement slowly. If you took five grams four times daily, and then maybe dropped it to half that dosage as a maintenance, that would be enough.

One of the main downsides to creatine is that, in order to take enough to be effective in the gym, sometimes this can cause a water holding problem. So water retention can blur muscular definition as the water is held or retained just under the skin. Usually by taking enough water during the workout and the rest of the day, as we'll come on to when we do the diet plan, this usually offsets this problem. It has been suggested that taking creatine in its ethyl ester form helps to guard against this and also improves the absorption of creatine by surrounding it with an ester. This ethyl ester form is also in an easy to take capsule, or tablet form. Since its launch just a few years ago, there have been many claims by supplement companies that this is the revolutionary creatine to take and is far superior to creatine monohydrate. However, more research needs to be done to substantiate these claims. If it's down to cost, then creatine monohydrate wins out overall and is proven to be very effective taken with other constituents of an ideal pre workout drink, beta alanine and citrulline.

Beta alanine is the building block of carnosine, a molecule that helps reduce the over-acidity of muscles. It also increases physical performance within the 60 to 240 second range. It can also aid a lean mass and appears to be a powerful antioxidant and antiaging compound. Similarly, citrulline is an amino acid which is turned into L-arginine. Citrulline supplementation is a more effective method of increasing L-arginine levels in the body than just purely by L-arginine alone. It's used in sports performance and used as a cardiovascular health supplement. It reduces fatigue and improves endurance in both aerobic and anaerobic prolonged exercise. L-citrulline also converts to arginine and increases ornithine levels in the plasma. This improves the ammonia recycling process and nitric oxide production. This helps to improve blood flow in muscles and is also used to alleviate erectile dysfunction caused by high blood pressure. Sometimes an added stimulant such as caffeine is added to pre workout drinks. It should be noted that with the pre workout drink the sugar solution should be no more than six percent. This is so that it allows quick emptying from the stomach and it won't be swishing around your inside while you're working out, and also so that we don't encourage a crash due to a fast insulin stimulation during the workout. Having a sugar solution less than six percent will allow you to rehydrate more readily which is important because if you include a stimulant such as caffeine this causes a dehydration effect.

Post Workout Drink

The main aim of the post workout drink is to replenish glycogen in the muscle, stimulate insulin to encourage a drive of both glucose and amino acids into the cells, to help to provide energy for protein synthesis to occur, and also provide the substrate for protein synthesis to occur. This means the drink must contain at least 50 grams of simple sugars such as glucose and also to contain a pre-digested or hydrolysed whey protein containing enough branched chain amino acids to improve this protein synthesis and also to include peptide bonded glutamine. We've discussed previously the benefits of glutamine in rehydrating and replenishing glycogen in the cells and also improving this anti-catabolic or anabolic response. There is an area of contention in sports nutrition circles regarding this so-called one hour window of opportunity for protein synthesis following a workout. After studying more than 80 articles, the consensus of opinion came down on the side that it is important to encourage taking in this post workout drink within the one hour window following a workout. V Kumar et al, from the Journal of Applied Physiology in 2009, did a study on the breakdown and synthesis of muscle protein during and after exercise. Muscle protein synthesis (MPS) and muscle protein breakdown (MPB) were both either unchanged or slightly depressed during exercise. However, after exercising when blood sugar levels were low, they were both greatly increased. Net protein muscle balance only became positive when amino acids were available. However, MPB was prevented mostly by insulin which was stimulated by glucose ingestion following the workout. Therefore, for maximum protein synthesis and minimum protein breakdown the amino acids and glucose from an available source of post workout drink need to be available and this maximum response is achieved after 30 minutes.

From the inflammatory process of muscle, following heavy resistance training, the levels of MPS and MPB remain elevated not for 48 hours but right up to consolidation remodelling by satellite cells four or five days later. So the take-home message here is that maximum protein synthesis and muscle breakdown occurs 30 minutes to one hour after the workout, but also lasts up to four to five days after. So it's important to get the right fast nutrition in and then followed by long term nutrition for the next four or five days to improve the chance of the muscle growing and getting stronger. Regarding this post workout inflammation it's been proven that slight inflammation is needed to produce enough satellite cells to stimulate this adaptive response. If we take anti-inflammatories in immediately following the workout, these interfere with and inhibit satellite cell production. If you do take anti-inflammatories, for whatever reason, do so only occasionally and well before a workout. Similarly, regarding antioxidants, these shouldn't be taken immediately following a workout as they can also affect regrowth stimuli and also insulin sensitivity. So leave antioxidants such as vitamin C and E alone following a workout. The reason for this is that production of free radicals through muscle damage during a workout is needed to stimulate optimum growth. The exact mechanisms are yet to be verified but it's likely that these free radicals switch on anabolic responses in the nuclei of muscle satellite cells involved in muscle re-proliferation. Mopping up these free radicals by using antioxidants is likely to lessen this anabolic response.

Micronutrients

The ingestion of micronutrients in the diet is very important to try and control all the enzymic activities of the body and it's important to prevent too much oxidative stress also. These come in the form of vitamins, minerals, antioxidants and trace elements. I'll go through a list of supplements that are required on the diet plan later on. If we think about the most essential antioxidants that we need to take in, these are vitamin E, vitamin C, coenzyme Q10 and selenium. Antioxidants are the cells defence system to protect the cell membranes and enzymes against free radical damage. Free radicals are highly reactive molecules which are produced from oxygen metabolism. Free radicals are like shrapnel attacking cells on the constituents, causing cell dysfunction or death. This is known as oxidative stress. Their main targets are lipids or fats, membranes, DNA, RNA and protein. Literature implicates free radicals in nearly every disease and pathological process. There are a small number, however, that are necessary for the synthesis of

159

substances such as hormones and they're also important in the body's immune system. As these antioxidants mop up these damaging free radicals, they're essential for good health. A deficiency in the body of these antioxidants and trace elements is detrimental to the health and sports performance, and leads to an increased incidence of oxidative stress. Although there is little data to substantiate the need for athletes to supplement, it is thought that an antioxidant supplement of 100 percent of the RDA on top of a well-balanced diet should provide an adequate insurance policy and be deemed relatively safe. Chronically elevated antioxidant levels could be detrimental to the positive aspect of free radicals, i.e. in immunity.

Berberine

The only other supplement that I want to mention which has recently come to light is Berberine. Berberine is an alkaloid extracted from various plants and used in traditional Chinese medicine. It's supplemented for its anti-inflammatory and antidiabetic effects. It can also improve intestinal health and lower cholesterol levels. Berberine is able to reduce glucose production in the liver. Human and animal research demonstrates that 1500 milligrams of Berberine taken in three doses of 500 milligrams each is as equally effective as taking 1500 milligrams of Metformin or 4 milligrams of Glibenclamide, two pharmaceutical drugs for treating Type II diabetes. Due to its normalising effect on blood sugar levels, especially taken after a meal, it can also help with body fat loss and insulin sensitivity. One of the main problems with ingesting carbohydrates as we get older is that we have a lowered insulin sensitivity, i.e. the glucose doesn't get driven into the cell and hangs around in the bloodstream causing problems. The Berberine improves this sensitivity and allows the insulin to be more effective. The only problem noted with Berberine is that it does tend to interact with certain medications such as antibiotics, and these can cause problems for the heart. So as long as people are careful that they don't take Berberine supplements along with antibiotics then there are no other known side effects from the use of this naturally occurring product.

160

Ketogenic Diets

It's a recent craze in bodybuilding circles for people to go on Ketogenic diets leading up to a bodybuilding or a physique contest. Ketosis is one of the most severe metabolic mistakes in protein synthesis and utilisation, including muscle mass accumulation, amino acid uptake, brain function and fat burning. The word ketosis comes from the root word ketones, which are compounds produced in the liver through the incomplete breakdown of fat. When the body is running out of carbohydrates or glucose, fats produce glucose themselves by the process of gluconeogenesis. This is under the mediation of the hormone called glucagon which is stimulated to do this when blood sugar levels are low. Fatty acids also convert to Acetyl-CoA in low glucose situations into ketones which are a slow energy producer. Amino acids can also be broken down into ketones or glucose for energy. If your goal is to reduce brain capacity and function whilst increasing body fat and decreasing lean muscle mass then ketosis is the answer.

Many protein products boast that they don't contain carbohydrates but this is metabolic suicide for protein metabolism and homeostasis (the normal state of the body). Proteins without carbohydrates causes a ketogenic state in humans which reduces the ability of the human body to create maximum muscle mass. Contrary to popular opinion, carbohydrates are required in protein synthesis and maintaining a regular dietary intake of non-insulin stimulating carbohydrates combined with protein prevents the protein from being used as an energy source and allows it to be available as building blocks to improve lean muscle mass. An adequate supply of these carbohydrates prevents the degradation of skeletal muscle and other tissues broken down into constituent amino acids and oxidised for energy. Combining protein and carbohydrates allows this gluconeogenesis to slow down, allowing amino acids to be freed. More importantly, it prevents ketosis. To prevent dietary ketosis you would need to consume at least 50 grams of carbohydrate per day, and when ingesting dietary protein, include an appropriate ratio of protein to carbs, which improves protein synthesis. High protein and low carbohydrate diets slow down metabolism. This causes a weight loss to occur in the muscle tissue as well as the fat tissue. When muscle mass is reduced in humans in response to ketosis, fat burning slows down and metabolic rate decreases. Ironically, this results in an increase in body fat and a decrease in muscle mass. Decreases in lean muscle mass cause the resting metabolic rates to decrease, since skeletal muscle requires more energy at rest than fat tissue. Fats can only be metabolised or burned when there is an adequate amount of glucose from carbohydrates present. Since fatty acids are degraded directly to Acetyl-CoA, they cannot be used as an energy source and can be transformed into ketones. These ketones are only meant to be used in a survival situation so ketosis is really a survival strategy for the body to slow down the catabolism of synthesising bodily proteins for energy by converting ketones to produce ATP in the absence of glucose. Glucose is still the preferred energy source for brain and muscle activity. Red blood cells cannot utilise ketones and they obviously, then, cannot supply oxygen to muscles. This being the case, after a few days of the muscle being sustained by the ketosis it then eventually starts to break down through catabolism. Added to this, ketones cause acidosis in the blood, so the blood will be more acidic than normal. This causes the kidneys to work harder to maintain the homeostasis of the body. So all in all, the body is in a serious stressful situation and the muscles in a serious catabolic or torn down state.

DIET PLAN 1

Typical off-season plan for a 200lb. bodybuilder who burns 2500- calories a day.
This would average out at 200g. protein, 300g. carbs, 50-70g. fat.
Protein and fat intake stays the same

DAY	Carb intake (g.)	Fluid intake (l.)	Day	Carb intake (g.)	Fluid intake (l.)	Day	Carb intake (g.)	Fluid intake (l.)
1	50	4	11	200	4	21	200	4
2	75	4	12	650	6	22	250	4
3	100	4	13	550	5	23	300	5
4	600	6	14	450	5	24	350	5
5	500	5	15	200	4	25	400	5
6	400	5	16	700	7	26	450	5
7	200	4	17	600	6	27	500	5
8	600	6	18	500	5	28	550	5
9	500	5	19	100	4	29	600	6
10	400	5	20	150	4	30	650	7

Correct Off-Season Diet Plan

If we look at the diet plan one, it shows a typical off-season plan for a 200lb bodybuilder who normally burns 2,500 calories a day. So this would average out at at least 200 grams of protein, 300 grams of carbs and about 70 grams of fat. So if we keep the protein and the fat intake the same, as you can see, we will then cycle the carbs. As we go through days one to ten, carbohydrate levels slowly increase and we get to a peak of about 600, and then it starts to drop again and then we peak at 600 again. The reason for this is to increase his metabolism so that he burns more than that 2,500 calories a day, but also provides more carbohydrate for protein synthesis. Notice his fluid intake also increases as his carbohydrate levels go up. For each gram of carbohydrate we need at least three grams of water, and then we also need to allow for respiration during the day and various enzymic activities that require water. So you can see he's peaking on six litres per day. When we go on to days 11 to 20, you notice then that his carbohydrate levels drop and peak a little bit higher than they did the first ten days. Again, we're trying to stimulate his metabolism. So he peaks at 700 grams on day 16 with a seven litre intake of water. As we go on then from days 21 you can see that his carbohydrate levels have dropped and they're very slowly increasing again. So at the end of this 30 day cycle, he's gone through a period of peaks and troughs with his carbohydrates, mainly so that he has enough carbohydrate to synthesise proteins, but then he doesn't overspill causing too much fat retention. So the main aim is to accumulate muscle mass without accumulating fat mass, and by cycling the carbs in this manner we achieve this.

If we go now to the Off-Season Micros in supplement form. All the supplements we've previously discussed, as in the antioxidants, like vitamin E, selenium, coenzyme Q10 and vitamin C (as you can see I tend to give examples of the Solgar make which I consider to be the highest standard.) The multivitamin mineral is called the VM-2000 which is also manufactured by Solgar. Some of the other supplements I didn't discuss earlier are, CLA, which helps to metabolise fatty acids when on a calorie restricted diet. So he's on this especially for the lower carbohydrate days. Also included is green tea,

Off season micro's in supplements

Supplement	Daily dose
Multivit/mineral (e.g. VM2000)	1
EPA/GLA (e.g. Solgar)	1
Esterised Vitamin C (e.g. Solgar)	1 x 2
Co-enzyme Q10 (60 mg)	1 x 2
Selenium (200 mg)	1
Vitamin E (1000 IU)	1
CLA (conjugated linoleic acid)	2g x 2
Green tea 400 mg	1 x 2
Vitamin D3 (1000 IU)	2
Creatine – ethyl ester (take 4 weeks on, 2 weeks off)	2g x 2
Berberine 400 mg	1 x 3
Niacin 500 mg	1 before training
Calcium / magnesium (e.g. Solgar ultimate bone support)	1 x 2

Pre contest micro's in supplements

Supplement	Daily dose
Multivit/mineral (e.g. VM2000)	1
EPA/GLA (e.g. Solgar)	1 x 2
Esterised Vitamin C (e.g. Solgar)	1 x 3
Co-enzyme Q10 (60 mg)	1 x 2
Selenium (200 mg)	1
Vitamin E (1000 IU)	1
CLA (conjugated linoleic acid)	2g x 2
Green tea 400 mg	2 x 2
Vitamin D3 (1000 IU)	2
Creatine – ethyl ester (take 4 weeks on, 2 weeks off)	2g x 2
Berberine 400 mg	Up to 6/day
Niacin 500 mg	1 before training
Calcium / magnesium (e.g. Solgar ultimate bone support)	1 x 2
Fat burners (see section on)	

which is a powerful antioxidant and also assists in metabolism as well. Vitamin D3 is added, especially during the winter months because we can suffer from a lack of sunlight and this country suffers from rickets unnecessarily so because we don't supplement this. Vitamin D3 is also important for testosterone production. The only other supplement there is the Niacin which acts as a nitric oxide stimulator and a vasodilator, it's naturally occurring in vitamin B and also the calcium and magnesium to prevent any cramping and also for normal function of the nervous system and bone density. Finally, on the off-season diet, although I've not given specific diets with the food set out, I've given you an indication of the type of foods you need to be eating for the protein sources and the carbohydrates sources, and the fat sources as well. What I've not mentioned in detail is the fact that we need to include fibre and greens into the diet. It's essential that we have at least 30 grams of fibre per day. These can be found from such dietary sources as grain products, pectins in fruits and cellulose in vegetables. Sometimes, some of the wheat based products produce a course fibre which can sometimes irritate the colon, and as most of us are susceptible to wheat intolerance I tend to indicate wherever possible to try gluten free sources. In some situations it might be necessary to supplement your fibre, in which case I recommend psyllium husk. This is a fine dietary fibre that actually cleanses the colon as well. With the greens, look for bean, pea, asparagus, spinach, kale and cabbage products.

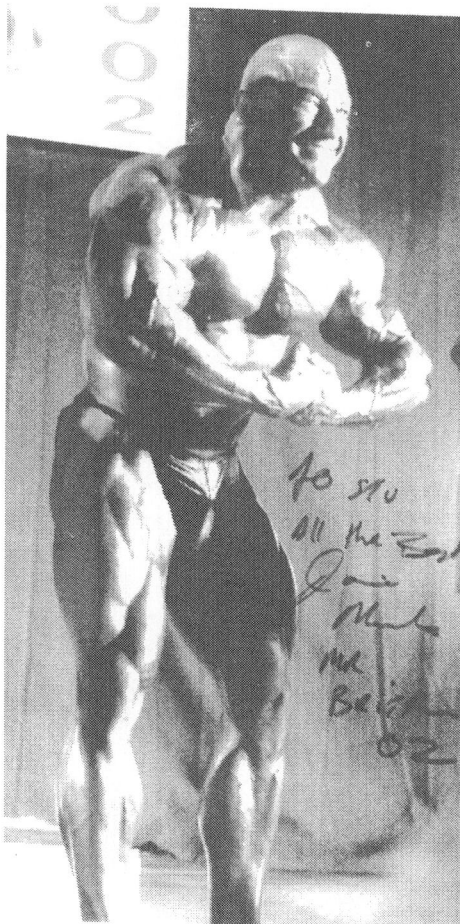

Jamie Manuel: Winner of the NABBA Universe
and British Titles. I am proud to have helped
Jamie through some very traumatic injuries!

DIET PLAN 2

Pre-contest diet example for a 200lb. lean bodybuilder going from 10% bodyfat to 4%
Protein and fat intake remains the same at 200g. and 50-70g. respectively.
This diet would be started 4-6 months prior to the event. Assuming this bodybuilder's
bodyweight has stayed the same on average 300g carb

DAY	Carb intake (g.)	Fluid intake (l.)	Day	Carb intake (g.)	Fluid intake (l.)	Day	Carb intake (g.)	Fluid intake (l.)
1	200	4	11	100	4	21	250	5
2	200	4	12	200	4	22	275	5
3	200	4	13	100	4	23	300	5
4	400	5	14	100	4	24	325	5
5	200	4	15	100	4	25	350	5
6	200	4	16	200	4	26	375	5
7	200	4	17	150	4	27	400	5
8	400	5	18	175	4	28	450	6
9	100	4	19	200	4	29	500	6
10	100	4	20	225	5	30	600	7

DIET PLAN 3

LAST 14 DAYS TO COMPETITION
Fat intake 50-70g daily. Supplements EGA, GLA (omega 3/6)

Day	Carbs (g.)	Fluid (l.)	Protein (g.)	Weights	Fat Burn	Fat Burners	Berb-erine	Vit C	GLA 2g. x 2	Low salt	Dandelion Root	Ethyl Ester Creatine
1	50	4	220	Yes	Yes ↑	Yes	0	2-3g.	Yes	Yes		2g. x 2
2	50	4	220	On	Yes ↑	Yes	0	2-3g.	Yes	Yes		2g. x 2
3	50	4	220	Split	Yes ↑	Yes	0	2-3g.	Yes	Yes		2g. x 2
4	1000	7	200	System	No	No	6	2-3g.	Yes	Yes		2g. x 2
5	1000	7	200	"	No	No	6	2-3g.	Yes	Yes but →		2g. x 2
6	200	7	200	"	Moderate	Yes	2	2-3g.	Yes	→		2g. x 2
7	250	7	200	"	Moderate	Yes	2	2-3g.	Yes	→		2g. x 2
8	300	7	200	"	Moderate	Yes	3	2-3g.	Yes	Low		2g. x 2
9	350	7	200	"	Moderate	Yes	3	2-3g.	Yes	Low		2g. x 2
10	400	7	200	"	No	No	4	2-3g.	Yes	Low		2g. x 2
11	450	6	200	No weights	No	No	5	2-3g.	Yes	Low	Yes ←	
12	500	5	200	No weights	No	No	6	2-3g.	Yes	Low	Yes ←	
13	50	4	400	No weights	No	No	2	6g.	Yes	0	Yes ←	
14	Show Day – it doesn't matter if you have eggs, steak etc. for breakfast as long as you have at least 4 hours before you are due onstage. Keep your low salt / seasoning out at this meal. For the next few hours, protein intake does not matter. Carb intake should be kept to low glycaemic carbs such as rice cakes which are easy on the stomach and don't give an insulin spike. Just 30g. carbs per hour will keep blood sugar levels normal.												

Fluid 1.5l. water, 80g glycerol, 6g vit C, 10 dandelion capsules, lemon juice, sip 300ml. per hour

169

Pre Contest Diet Plan

Pre Contest Diet Mistakes

1. Not leaving enough time to lose the body fat before a competition.
2. Keeping carbohydrates too low for too long and not cycling them.
3. Eating too much protein and also the wrong type at the wrong time.
4. Using ketogenic diets with a high fat content.
5. (although technically not dietary) Dropping poundages and increasing reps and sets before a show.
6. Not drinking enough water both prior to and near to the show.
7. Eating sugary carbs near to and on competition day.
8. Over-manipulation of potassium and sodium levels.
9. Not eating enough fibre and greens.

Macros

Although the macros for proteins and fats technically don't change from that of the off-season diet, we can allow some manipulation nearer to the competition. The main thing to be manipulated, as we'll see on the dietary plans, is the carbohydrates. With regard to the macros, the same thing applies to the pre contest diet as did the off-season diet. If we look through the pre contest macro list for supplements we can see that it's essentially the same as the off-season diet. The only difference is that the Berberine is increased only on high carbohydrate diet days up to six a day in split dosages, so that's two taken three times a day. The only other inclusion is the fat burners right at the bottom of the supplement page. After some searching and analysing of various products for fat burning I managed to find a fat burner called Lipodrene from Hi-Tech Pharmaceuticals in the US. This is the strongest legal fat burner today. The use of ephedrine is illegal to take and sell as a drug but ephedra extract is a healthier, legal form without the alkaloids associated with ephedrine. It wasn't that low doses of ephedrine were dangerous, it's just that as usual this substance was abused and it caused it to be banned in 2004. Lipodrene has the right balance of ephedra extract and other botanics but I also recommend that you take aspirin along with the Lipodrene to potentiate the effect of the ephedra as a fat burner. If this is the case, then take enteric coated aspirin (75 milligrams), along with the Lipodrene, twice daily. Be careful with organisations that drug test for caffeine as higher than normal levels may cause them some concern. Even taking cough medicine in the IOC governed sports can cause you problems without a medical prescription. If we move on to look at the table Diet Plan Two, we can see that this is a pre contest diet for a 200lb lean bodybuilder going from a ten percent body fat to a four percent body fat, hopefully. This needs to be started four to six months prior to the event. We can see that protein and fat intake remain the same, at 200 grams, and 70 grams of fat respectively. Now, from days one to ten, we can see it's basically a three low, one high carbohydrate fluctuation. So it's going from 200 grams and then doubling on the fourth day and back down to 200 again. This is repeated but halving the levels of carbs. So we peak out at a low of 100 grams on the 15th day. Then on the 16th day onwards we slowly, incrementally increase the carbs by 25 grams per day. We then peak at 600 on the 30th day. This serves two purposes;

1. To speed up the metabolism so more fat burning can occur, and;

2. To replenish glycogen levels in the muscle so the muscle can be maintained or even small gains could be made towards the last third of the month.

It's not unknown for people to be still losing body fat on the 25th day of the month with only five days to go to start the plan again. So they can end up really lean and full by the 30th day. This diet plan can then be repeated going back to day one again, and you repeat this cycle right up until the last 14 days before the competition.

This moves us on to Diet Plan Three. Here you can see that we've listed the 14 days up to competition. We've got the carbs, the fluid levels, the protein intake and then also when to do the

171

weights and when not to do the weights. So you can see in the last four days, or the last three days before the competition, no weights are done on those days, and we allow the carbohydrates to seep into the system. Notice that the heaviest carbs are done on the week prior to the show and then we're kind of coast in then so that we don't cause any water retention and we don't drastically have to resort to diuretic usage. The only naturally occurring diuretics that probably assist us is the dandelion root on the last three days.

You can see that we use Lo Salt in the diet, which is something you can get from the supermarket which is higher in potassium than sodium and helps to maintain sodium levels to a minimum but not to go so low as to upset homeostasis of the body. Creatine supplements are taken right up until the last four days which could possibly hold some water, and we fat burn, as in doing low intensity aerobics, quite a lot on the week prior to the week of the competition, but no fat burning on the last four days to allow those carbohydrates to replenish the glycogen in the muscle, and no excess carbohydrates are burnt off. We even stop the fat burners then just to make sure that the body's metabolism can slow down and we can seep those carbohydrates into the muscle to create as much fullness as possible. You'll notice from days 12 to 13 we drastically cut the carbs and double the protein. We also increase vitamin C and also we utilise the dandelion root. This all acts as a natural diuretic effect but without losing intramuscular water. So the water comes completely from under the skin. By increasing the protein level, the kidneys try and flush out any excess water because it increases amino acid levels in the blood and creates an increase in nitrogen which is then passed out with a natural diuretic response.

Come the show day, we make sure that we don't do anything drastic and we continue to rehydrate the body, albeit with slightly lower levels of water, taking 1.5 litres in over a few hours. We continue with the vitamin C, six grams, and the dandelion capsules in the lemon juice. So we're sipping about 300 millilitres per hour. The only other thing to introduce is something called glycerol. You might have seen Glycerol in pharmacy shops as a cough suppressant but, technically, it's a sugar alcohol and it has a super hydrating effect, drawing on water to increase blood volume. It can rehydrate over and above that of taking water in alone but also without any water retention. Due to its blood volume increase, when taken prior to a competition it can have two effects. Any intramuscular dehydration can be corrected to give the muscle a fuller look, and increases in blood plasma can increase vascularity. I recommend not taking more than one gram per kilogram of lean body weight or it can upset your stomach. It's best to try it a couple of weeks prior to the show to make sure that you can tolerate it. So for a 90 kilogram bodybuilder, lean, he would take 70 to 80 grams in and 1.5 litres of water, and he'd take this for a couple of hours prior to going onstage.

Chapter 10 – Off-Season and Pre Contest Diet Plans – Summary

1.   Thinking about your macros, don't eat too much protein and also don't eat the wrong type at the wrong time. In other words, complete proteins during the day and more simple hydrolysed whey proteins post workout.

2.   Take your carbohydrate sources as mainly complex during the day and simple post workout and also cycle your carbs during your diet, whether it be for muscle gain or fat loss.

3.   Don't use ketogenic diets whatsoever. They don't work and they should not be in the arsenal of a competitive bodybuilder.

4.   Make sure you have adequate fluids during the day, preferably in the form of bottled water, rather than fizzy pop. If it has to be fizzy pop make sure that it's a diet version. So on high carbohydrate days up to six or seven litres per day, depending on your body weight.

5.   Ensure your fat intake is from a number of sources. Try and shift your Omega-6 to 3 balance to two-one (2:1). Your fat sources should come from various nuts, oils, coconut oil and oily fish.

6.   On pre contest dieting make sure that you leave enough time to lose the fat before the competition. If you're over twelve percent, four to six months may be necessary.

7.   In the off-season diet, make sure you don't bulk up or ingest too many calories over a long period of time.

8.   Don't ingest too much of the wrong types of fats, i.e. trans fats and animal saturated fats.

9.   Make sure on both pre and off-season diets that you eat adequate greens and fibre, including psyllium husk as a supplement for the fibre.

10.   Make sure the post workout drink has adequate simple sugars and also hydrolysed whey, and is taken within 30 minutes of the workout.

11.   Make sure you eat at least six meals a day spaced out every three hours and also spreading your protein intake out fairly evenly as well as carbs.

12.   When taking antioxidants, make sure you base your intake around vitamin E, vitamin C, coenzyme Q10 and selenium, but don't take your antioxidants straight after a workout.

13.   If you decide to take a pre workout drink, make sure that it contains creatine, beta alanine, citrulline, caffeine and the sugar content is less than 6%.

When fat burning try to follow the fat burning example as shown in the table, so fat burning for either pre contest or even off-season should consist of low intensity long duration. So after 30 minutes your body is burning fat as an energy rather than carbohydrates providing you're only working at ten percent of your VO2 max. As a rough guide, most people's heart rate shouldn't go above 120. You can see there that working at a higher VO2 max, that the calories burnt are 1,000, but you can see that 90 percent of the calories are coming from carbohydrates and only ten percent from fats. So even though 1,000 calories have been burnt you've used a lot of your carbohydrates out of your muscles, or instead in that one hour, if you only work at ten percent of your VO2 max, for most people that's about a 120 heart rate, you can see there that although 500 calories have been burnt, 90 percent of those have been fat.

Fat Burning Example

In 1 hour

10% VO2 max 500 cals burnt 10% carbs 90% fat = 450 cals fat burn
100% VO2 max 1000 cals burnt 10% fat 90% carbs fat = 100 cals

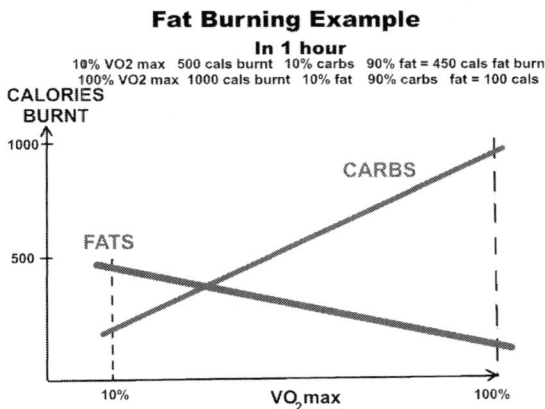

CALORIES BURNT

1000

CARBS

FATS

500

10% VO_2 max   100%

175

CHAPTER 11
ERGOGENIC AIDS

In the context of sport, an ergogenic aid can be broadly defined as a technique or substance used for the purpose of enhancing performance. They may be legal or illegal. They can be pharmacological, physiological, psychological or nutritional.

For the purposes of this book, we will not debate the moral issues as to whether the taking of certain ergogenics is classed as cheating. We, however accept that these substances will be used by individuals seeking an advantage. The aim of this chapter is to point out the pro's and con's of their use and if they are to be used, how to do it more safely! I feel it a duty to point out the health issues that can be generated by misuse of some ergogenics. We will concentrate mainly on the nutritional and pharmacological aids rather than go into other areas such as motivational and psychological aids. Some physiological aids such as Hyperbaric and Cryogenic chambers may have their uses to aid recovery, but we will concentrate on anabolic type aids.

NATURAL ERGOGENICS

a) Creatine
b) Testosterone Boosters
c) Growth Hormone Boosters
d) Berberine

Above are listed the main ergogenics that have been verified to be highly productive when it comes to gaining muscle and strength. There are a lot of other legal supplements that have been purported to be good ergogenic aids, but under strict scientific study these fall down. If you want to cut through all the hype and check properly if a supplement's claims have been substantiated or not, then go on to examine.com on the internet . This is an independant body of experts who identify any peer reviewed articles in scientific journals on various products. They form an informed opinion as to its effectiveness. A lot of the amino acids and vitamins have been covered in the previous chapter, including Creatine and Berberine, so we will concentrate on the others in the list.

Testosterone Boosters

Testosterone is the most important male sex hormone, also called androgens. The body uses cholesterol to manufacture androgens. The androgens are produced in the testes. The final product is testosterone which fulfils 2 main functions in the male:

1) Development of the male sexual characteristics such as deepening of the voice, hair growth, increased production by sebaceous glands, development of the penis, sexual behaviour and libido. It is also involved in the maturation of sperm. These are called the Androgenic functions of Testosterone. Men distinguish themselves from women by the amount of testosterone they produce daily. men produce on average between 4-10 mg and women 0.15-0.4 mg daily.

2) The second main function of testosterone is the promotion of Protein Synthesis. This promotes a high anabolic or 'building up' situation. Faster muscle protein turnover, synthesis of new cellular proteins, faster recovery from exercise, injury or illness and increases in red blood cells are all achieved. The entire metabolism and an increase in fat burning is also increased.

Despite a wealth of Testosterone Boosters available on the market, when examined under scrutiny, very few of them give an appreciable rise in free testosterone. Only 2 supplements are available that stand up to peer review as to appreciably increase natural testosterone levels. These are Vitamin D3 and Zinc. Zinc deficiency in the diet can hinder natural testosterone production. By increasing your daily intake of zinc, you can appreciably push up your own testosterone production. Zinc comes naturally from shellfish.

Another vitamin which increases manufacture of testosterone in the body is vitamin D, especially Vitamin D3. If you can increase vitamin D3 levels up to and over 3000 IU daily, this increases serum testosterone by a substantial amount. The RDA for vitamin D is only 400-600 IU daily and is easily available from food sources such as oily fish such as mackerel and salmon, dairy products, and egg yolks. Supplementation may be required to get your levels to a stage where testosterone is boosted adequately.

Exercise

The right type of exercise also helps to stimulate the production of testosterone in the body. Providing the exercise is of high enough resistance and intensity to cause slight damage to the muscle, this stimulatory response causes the Pituitary gland to produce more LH (Luteinising hormone) and FSH (Follicle stimulating Hormone) which in turn cause the testes to release more testosterone. Similarly, when performing aerobic exercise, if the exercise is intense enough and of short duration, this also provides a stimulatory response. Long term endurance training can have the reverse effect!

Growth Hormone Boosters

Human Growth hormone is an anabolic 191sequence amino-acid polypeptide hormone. It is synthesised, stored and secreted by the somatotrophic cells of the pituitary gland in your brain. It stimulates mainly bone and muscle tissue growth through the metabolism of protein, fats and carbohydrates. It is also a strong regulator of immune function amongst other physiological processes. During early childhood and adolescence it is essential for promoting height. In adulthood, it is responsible for a number of maintenance tasks:

1) Keeping your body lean and reducing fat accumulation
2) Protecting and strengthening bones
3) Protecting internal organs from age related deterioration
4) Promoting more rapid nail and hair growth

178

5) Maintaining circulation and healthy cholesterol levels

The release of human growth hormone (HGH) from the pituitary gland is made by various physiological stimuli e.g. exercise, sleep, types of food intake. Like other hormones HGH works by interacting with specific receptor sites on the surface of cells. The HGH then activates anabolic processes within the target cell. Depending on the type of cell involved, different actions occur. For example; in muscle cells, HGH causes increased cell repair, division and proliferation. In liver cells, HGH stimulates the production of Insulin Growth Factor (IGF-1), which can then be taken up by cells such as muscle to initiate repair through protein synthesis. There are other isoforms of HGH released in other tissues such as FGF (fibroblastic growth factor) involved in regrowth of ligament and tendon tissue as well as MGF (Mechano Growth Factor). MGF is released directly in the muscle especially when the muscle is subjected to slow eccentric or negative resistance. This is one good reason to include slow eccentric training in your program as this growth factor improves protein synthesis and growth locally in the muscle that is stimulated. This slow contraction eccentrically also has benefits to the tendon structures as it also stimulates release of growth factors that initiate collagen production. Unfortunately HGH production starts to diminish almost exponentially from your 30's onwards. This leads to a potential reduction in lean bodymass and bone density, combined with an increase in bodyfat. This can also increase cardiovascular risk factors. In other words you quickly begin to look and feel older as HGH declines. This process of HGH deficit with age is called SOMATOPAUSE and tends to be overlooked in medical circles as a natural ageing process with no treatment administered. There are a number of actions we can take to offset this process to a degree. These will be dealt with in the next chapter. For the younger athlete, there are still some steps we can use to potentiate our natural production of HGH:

1) Increase the intensity of our training. With resistance training, this would be the more glycolytic type training. With aerobic training, it would be shortening the

179

activity time but increasing the load and performing it in intervals. e.g. Tabata style training. This training would ideally be done on a stationary bike, stepper, stairmaster, cross trainer or concept 2 rower. Intervals should be kept short, with little rest between e.g. 20secs on,10secs off for 8 cycles! This is not for the faint hearted and will absolutely burn your muscles and lungs like never before if done maximally! This will boost these growth hormone isoforms and is more conducive to bodybuilding than long ,drawn out aerobic sessions! If this is done 3 times a week, it will boost your lactate reabsorption, anaerobic threshold, maximum oxygen uptake, Growth hormone response, capillary network in muscles and overall cardiovascular efficiency!

2) <u>Getting enough sleep.</u> Sleep is a massive stimulus for the Growth hormone axis. Making sure you get 7-8 hours per night with a 15 or 20 minute power nap during the day will maximise this response as well as helping your immune system and stress levels. When you sleep, you go through several cycles, from light sleep where you wake relatively easily to heavy sleep where you are soundly asleep and much harder to wake up from. During stages 3 and 4 of your slow wave sleep cycle is when you release most of your HGH during the night.

3) <u>Arginine.</u> The amino acid L-Arginine has been proven to be effective at releasing HGH when taken on an empty stomach 30 mins before retiring at night. Arginine needs a safe pathway to cross the blood brain barrier and Dr Ann de Wees Allen from the Glycaemic Research Institute in Washington developed a cell signalling Blind Amino acid Rider to help transport the Arginine in the form of a fruit Glycoside. This also makes it more palatable to take in drink form. This allows the arginine to produce more GHRF (Growth Hormone Releasing Factor). This supplement was originally called Tri Matrix, then developed by a company called Synergy into ProArgi 9. This also

combines it with L-Citrulline to help potentiate the effect and Vitamins K, C and D3 which all act together synergistically to maximise nitric oxide production as well. This is very important for circulatory and vascular structures as we will see in the next chapter. All the amino acids used by Synergy are of the purest pharmaceutical grade which is very important as you do not want contaminants distorting the positive effects. As such PROARGI 9 is the ONLY supplement listed in the Physicians Desk Reference Manual , recommended for use by doctors. Proargi 9 comes in 5g sachets, but 10g is needed to get a good HGH response.

UNNATURAL ERGOGENICS

Anabolic Steroids/ Testosterone

Anabolic and Androgenic steroids are synthetically manufactured compounds which are similar in structure to the male hormone testosterone. They are therefore defined as synthetic derivatives of testosterone. The main intention in developing these compounds was to increase the anabolic effect and decrease the androgenic effect when compare to testosterone. It would maximise protein synthesis but without the masculising secondary sexual characteristics of testosterone. Despite maximising their efforts to produce an anabolic only product, this was not achieved. So even the purest anabolic steroid has some of these effects. Some steroids have a stronger anabolic effect than testosterone and some have a weaker one. They are taken orally or injected intramuscularly. The injections pass into the blood stream almost immediately, whereas the orals have to go through the digestive tract before reaching the liver. From here, the substance is wholly or partially broken down and sent onto the blood stream. Once in the blood stream, it attaches to specific donor cells i.e. muscle cells. Here in the muscle cell, it bonds to a receptor site which then transmits the information to the cell nucleus where a transcription takes place.   RNA (Ribonucleic Acid) then leaves the nucleus, where a translation takes place and protein synthesis

181

increases within the cell. Another advantage of anabolic steroids is they increase the phosphocreatine synthesis (creatine) in the muscle cell. As you remember from earlier chapters, this in the initial explosive energy required by the muscle during intense work. The rest of the steroid molecule passes back into the blood stream where it is either eliminated by the body or it is converted into the female sex hormone oestrogen. This process is called aromatisation. The body uses various enzymes to perform this change. The body can also convert the molecule into DHT or Dihydrotestosterone. DHT shows a higher affinity to receptor sites in muscle than testosterone does which results in a much higher potential for protein synthesis and growth. DHT can also attach itself to hair follicle receptors and can cause premature hair loss in steroid users.

Side effects. As with any drug, any overdosing or overuse can lead to potential health damaging side effects. Although the misuse of steroids and growth hormones cannot be condoned, it is difficult to uninvent or stop the use of a product that has obvious performance enhancing capability. I personally cannot stop every athlete I advise from using them and so , if they are insisting on their use, I feel it necessary to guide them along the safest and healthiest road possible and never sacrifice their future health for the temporary success in their sport. I also advise certain blood tests that need to be done if this is to be the case. We will discuss these in depth in the next chapter. My advice would be to never 'go it alone'!! Never cycle these drugs without knowing what affect it is having on your body chemistry!! Seek out a reliable physician or qualified person to help you!

1) Inhibition of the Testicular Axis : When an anabolic or testosterone drug is taken over and above the natural production levels of the body, there comes a time, when the Testicular axis or normal testosterone cycle of production begins to shut down. This can have serious connotations. The Testicular axis table will be gone through in more detail in the next chapter, but suffice to say that testicular secretions will be reduced if this process of using an exogenous source of testosterone

continues. Initial symptoms include reduced testosterone production, increased oestrogen production resulting in loss of muscle, gaining fat, gynaecomastia of the nipple area (growth of breast tissue). Longer term shutdown can occur depending on the length of the dose cycle, the type of steroids used and the dosage. This can ultimately lead to cardiovascular problems, sterility, reduced sperm count, depression and libido loss. It is a mistaken belief that the taking of HCG (human chorionic gonadotrophin) and clomiphene can turn this situation around. Enough time needs to be given to allow the Testicular axis to reset. This is usually relative to the length of time the artificial hormones were administered. Its no use to come off for 6 weeks or so, as the endocrine system takes much longer to reset!. Occasionally spermatogenesis never restarts and athletes can be rendered permanently sterile!.

2) Water and Salt retention. Most steroids can cause an electrolyte imbalance within the body. This causes the storage of excess extracellular water and sodium. This causes a swelling of peripheral tissues (oedema). This can be tested for by pushing your thumb hard into the tissues round your ankle for 5 secs. If you indent more than a cm. then you are holding excess water. Water is also increased intracellularly which will indeed benefit the muscle tissue. The drawback is the increased water retention under the skin and in the blood. This can also elevate the athlete's blood pressure. The degree of this water retention depends on the type, dosage and length of duration of the steroid use. In order to combat this problem, then drink adequate amounts of water daily as water itself acts as a diuretic. Increase vitamin C, decrease salt intake, increase potassium intake, take a natural water eliminator such as Dandelion Root. Increasing potassium and decreasing relative sodium can be done by using ' Low Salt' as a condiment seasoner for food instead of salt.

3) <u>Gynaecomastia.</u> This occurs due to breast tissue growth in male athletes around the nipple area. It can also cause fatty deposits in this area. This is all due to the partial conversion of the steroid into the female hormone oestrogen. Its process is called Aromatisation. This may be avoided by using a steroid that has a zero or very low aromatisation. Also, by adding in an antioestrogen such as Nolvadex or Arimidex can treat the symptoms, but careful selection of anabolics sorts out the cause.

4) <u>Acne.</u> This is largely due to genetic predisposition and is due to receptor site affinity to DHT at the sebaceous glands. As you remember, anabolics are partially converted to DHT which has a strong affinity to muscle cells, but also to sebaceous glands. This leads to overproduction of sebum and blocks the pores. This leads to pimples, pustules and sometimes cysts. Treatment can be very successful with a combination of UVA A/B wavelengths combined with collagen forming Red Light therapy at approx 660nm wavelength. They have just brought out a combination tube for sunbeds incorporating all the correct wavelengths. It is the Collatan tube and we now use this in the clinic. When combined with drugs such as tetracycline and accutane, this can be even more effective at clearing acne altogether.

5) <u>Psychic changes.</u> Men and women undergoing long term use of steroids can show more aggressive behaviour. It usually depends on whether they have natural aggressive tendencies to start with, but anabolics can enhance these if they are already there. The benefit of this can be a better intensity in the gym, but the downside is an inability to cope with the general anxieties of life. These people can become easily irritated, quick tempered and intolerant.

6) <u>Gastrointestinal symptoms.</u> These symptoms are associated solely with the use of oral steroids. Some

184

people suffer from gastric overfullness, nausea, vomiting and diarrhoea. Sometimes tablets can be taken with meals to alleviate this. It is safer and less stressful on the liver to administer steroids by intramuscular injection.

7) <u>Baldness.</u> Male pattern balding can be caused through steroid use, where the individual has a strong affinity for DHT in the hair follicles. This causes the hair to fall out. Sometimes this hair loss is irreversible. In only seems to happen in those people who already have a genetic predisposition for hairloss.

8) <u>Cardiovascular defects.</u> Steroid use has also been linked with cardiovascular problems. A number of theories tend to put the blame on an elevated total cholesterol and triglyceride level caused by steroids increasing the chances of a cardiovascular incident. However, recent evidence does not go along with the elevation of cholesterol being directly linked to Heart Disease. There are many indigenous tribes around the world that have naturally high total cholesterol levels and an extremely low incidence of heart disease. (Check out the book 'The Great Cholesterol Con' by Dr Malcolm Kendrick). In this book, Kendrick lambasts a powerful pharmaceutical industry and an unquestioning medical community who, he claims perpetuate the madcap claims of 'Good' and 'Bad' cholesterol and cholesterol levels to convince millions of people to spend billions of pounds on statins causing an elevated level of stress and anxiety, which is the real cause of fatal heart disease!

The main problem to look out for with anabolic steroid usage is something called High Haematocrit. Anabolics increase the production of erythrocytes (Red blood Cells) which leads to an elevated Haematocrit or concentration of red cells in the blood. This in effect 'thickens' the blood increasing chances of clot formation and coronary artery obstruction which could lead to heart attacks. Other neck or cranial artery obstruction could lead to strokes.

Another main cause of strength athletes developing athero and arteriosclerosis is not cholesterol, but a substance called Homocysteine. Homocysteine is produced when anabolics metabolise in the body. A number of studies done in Exercise Physiology journals have proven that a large number of strength athletes suffering fatal heart attacks all had severe arteriosclerosis directly from High Homocysteine levels. Emboli from their damaged arteries caused their deaths as reported on their autopsies.

It must be stressed that regular blood tests should be done to check levels of Homocysteine and Haematocrit. In order to keep these levels under control, there are a number of natural products that may help.

Serrapeptase: This is a proteolytic enzyme derived from the silk worm. It helps to break down protein debris in the body including emboli and debris from arteriosclerosis in the form of a thrombus. The only problem is getting it into the system orally. It needs to be taken on an empty stomach.

Nattokinase   Another fibrinolytic enzyme is Nattokinase derived from the Japanese food Natto. It helps to break down the fibrin part of blood clots, thereby helping to prevent them forming.

Aspirin   Derived from White willow bark, Aspirin is one of the most underated drugs available. It acts as an anticoagulant, helping make the blood less viscous through platelet mobility. Although it sometimes gets bad press due to its tendency to cause stomach irritation and sometimes ulcers, in lower doses of 75mg, it can be taken daily as a failsafe for your blood viscosity. It also has an anti-inflammatory effect and has also been proven to guard against some cancers, especially colonic cancer. To make it even safer for the stomach, it can be obtained as an enteric coated tablet. I recommend all bodybuilders who are taking anabolics to seriously consider a daily dose of 75mg!

186

Recent studies have now shown that the application of LOW INTENSITY CONTINUOUS ULTRASOUND on major arteries such as Femoral and carotid can help to break down excess red blood cells (erythrocytes) and lower your haematocrit levels, making your blood less viscous and reducing your risk of blood clots. This can be done using a Therapeutic Ultrasound machine such as used by physiotherapists. The protocol required is 0.4 watts/cm2 continuous beam for 10 mins applied daily for 7 days.

Homocysteine Modulator: The supplement company, Solgar recognise the correlation between high homocysteine levels and cardiac disease, and as a result have produced this supplement. It contains Trimethyl glycine which mops up any excessive homocysteine in the blood.

So, in conclusion, for all bodybuilders to maintain good cardiovascular health and to protect against cardiac problems in the future, consider adopting the protocols mentioned above as well as regular blood checks. The blood test to ask your GP to do is an FBC (Full Blood Count). This will assess all your red and white blood cell levels. If you want to keep it private, then I suggest using a company called 'MEDICHECKS' who conduct private blood analysis and give you a report.

9)   Prostate Hypertrophy Most increases in size of the prostate gland is benign or non cancerous. This occurs naturally as we age. The term for this is BPH (Benign Prostatic Hypertrophy). Prostatic enlargement can affect urinary continence if it enlarges to a point that it presses on the bladder. This affects stretch receptors in the bladder, making you want to urinate more frequently. If the urine flow is reduced, the bladder doesn't always release its normal amount of urine and this can lead to bladder infections as the urine stagnates. If you need to go more than 4 times nightly and your flow is reduced, it is a sign the prostate may have enlarged.   As testosterone converts to DHT, the receptor sites in the prostate have an affinity for this.

187

DHT has been shown to cause prostatic enlargement. Some studies have shown that large doses of Saw Palmetto can help to reduce prostate size over a long period of time. (Taken consistently for at least 12 months). As the prostate gland grows, the level of the prostate specific antigen (PSA) also tends to increase. Some studies show that increased PSA levels may be connected with increase predisposition to prostate cancer. Other studies show that this is not necessarily the case and more factors are involved. Although doctors suggest a prostatic biopsy for men with high levels of PSA, this is fraught with more problems than they suggest. It is a very invasive and potentially damaging procedure which has been known to cause erectile dysfunction and urinary incontinence as well as pelvic inflammation and infection. There are other procedures to check for other protein markers in the urine to rule out cancer. Currently, though, these are only available privately. If the BPH is shown to be benign, it can be controlled and reduced with a drug called finasteride which blocks the DHT receptor sites.

10) Kidney Damage. The kidneys are under more stress during steroid usage. They are involved in the filtration of toxic by products of anabolic metabolism. High blood pressure and long term electrolyte imbalance can eventually lead to changes in kidney function. Maintaining good hydration is required to lessen the concentration of these toxic products. Along with increased stress on the kidneys, elevation of liver enzymes, especially non specific AST and ALT enzymes also occurs. These enzymes are also produced by the muscles under stress and often result in abnormally high levels. This should be taken into consideration when conducting tests on the strength athlete, as what is normal for them can be classed as abnormal for Joe Bloggs! As long as Bilirubin and Albumin Liver tests are normal in the strength athlete, there is unlikely to be any long term damage. I find this problem also occurs when strength athletes are given the standard kidney test

188

known as GFR. This measures the rate at which creatinine is released by the kidney, but is much different for the strength athlete. In USA , they have to deal with strength athletes regularly in American Football Associations and have perfected a multiplication factor to be applied to the GFR level to give a clearer reading for the kidney's efficiency. The ideal formula for GFR levels is the Cockcroft-Gault formula multiplied by 1.2.

Growth Hormone

Normal growth hormone production in a young mature male athlete will be less than 2IU daily. When athletes supplement this, doses of up to 16 IU per day have been reported. If this level of usage were sustained for any length of time, the side effects would be life changing! The most damaging effect potentially is LVH (Left ventricular Hypertrophy). Any athlete that has a high oxygen demand for his sport requires the heart to pump blood efficiently in high volumes and output. This therefore stresses the heart, and as with any muscle put under load, it will adapt by changing morphology. As a result, there is a 'normal' hypertrophy of the left venticle of the heart. This is the muscular part responsible for the final push of blood round the body. If, however, this hypertrophy enlarges too much, it affects the efficiency of the heart, and the muscle struggles to maintain this output for any length of time. This can result in all manner of associated problems such as backpressure, valve problems, congestion, etc. Other side effects such as carpal tunnel syndrome, where the median nerve in the wrist is compressed causing pain and numbness in the hand result from enhanced receptor sites in the connective tissues covering nerves resulting in overgrowth and pressure build up. Other tissues involved in overgrowth are bony tissues, resulting in increased exostosis of bones on the wrist, hands, feet and forehead. If cancerous tissues such as tumours have a strong affinity, these will increase in size also! As growth hormone affects blood sugar levels by increasing them sharply after use, it can in extended use lead to desensitisation of insulin, meaning it works less efficiently to drive blood sugars into the cells. This can lead to Diabetes. If

189

growth hormone is taken at all, it must be used when the blood sugars are low, ie in the morning before breakfast or after a workout. It must be emphasised that for the younger athlete, the taking of exogenous growth hormone will damage the Growth Hormone axis, resulting in a shutting down of the natural growth hormone response in long term usage.

In order to offset these effects, dosage should not be high and only taken for short periods of time e.g. 8 weeks. Use natural blood insulin sensitisers such as berberine and be careful when you administer. Of course my advice for any athlete under 40 is to go down the natural route if possible!

Growth Hormone Releasers

ProArgi 9+   The only natural Growth Hormone releaser I would recommend is ProArgi9 by Synergy. I have done a lot of research in this area as I feel it is important for me to advise athletes that work with me as effectively as I can without compromising health. In 1998, 3 scientists from America won a Nobel Prize for their work on Nitric Oxide being so important for cardio vascular heath. Following on from their formula, Dr Joe Prendergast and Dr Ann de Wees Allen devised an ideal formula for Nitric Oxide stimulation for a company called Synergy. Further studies uncovered other benefits including an up regulation of Growth hormone releasing factor when taken at doses of 10g before retiring. This has been recommended to treat Somatopause, a condition where natural growth hormone levels decline below a certain baseline level with age.   The 2 main blood factors which indicate somatopause are IGF-BP 3 and IGF-1 levels. When these fall below certain age related levels, then it is a strong indicator you are in Somatopause. The first line of defence is then to make sure quality of sleep, rest and exercise is in the right balance. Then the administering of ProArgi9 at 2 satchets per night for 6 months can result in a 30% increase in these levels. This can thus help to restore a more normal, natural hormone level.

Sermorelin.   Rather than immediately jumping to taking exogenous growth hormone as most strength athletes not under restrictions will do, why not check whether your natural releasing factors are down? Undergoing the above blood tests will give you an indication. This releasing factor is known as GHRH, but it can also be synthesised as a peptide called Sermorelin. This is administered by some Endocrine clinics in America rather than Growth Hormone to try to kick start the pituitary gland to produce increased Growth Hormone levels again. I would advise the use of the Proargi 9 product for 6 months first and then retesting. If levels are rising, then this should be adequate. The Sermorelin, sadly is unavailable through clinics in the UK, but Anti-ageing endocrine clinics in the USA have good results with it.

Other Peptides.   In the last few years, there has been a preponderance of 'so called labs' producing performance enhancing peptides. Many of these are unregulated and do not produce mass spectrometry or chromatograph studies to prove their products are legitimate. It is a black market produced alongside anabolic manufacture and you have no way of determining the sterile quality of the products. The Belgian Federal Agency for Products and Customs department are striving together with their global counterparts to curtail the trafficking of these products. Very often they are supplied in ampoules that are not labelled. Very often, just a white powder in the vial, without any reported certificate of authenticity. Most of these peptides produce by genuine labs are very light and temperature sensitive and have to be stored under rigidly strict conditions. Any variation from this can cause a denaturation of the product, rendering it useless! Although some encouraging results have been reported with these peptides on animals, not enough studies on humans have been done to prove safety and efficacy.

Genetics

Good genetics is the most effective Ergogenic aid you could have! Without good genetics, no matter how good your training and nutrition, your improvements would be limited, and the chances of being a top professional bodybuilder zero! Good genetics can come in varies forms and levels. We can break it down into the 3 following divisions: 1) SOMATOTYPE, 2) FIBRE-TYPE, 3) GENETIC MUTATED GENE'S (Myostatin and ACTN 3 Genes).

1) Somatotype: There are 3 main bodyshapes or somatotypes's, mesomorph, ectomorph and endomorph. People that are predominantly mesomorph have broad shoulders, increased muscle mass, low bodyfat and narrow hips. The ectomorph shape is slim or thin, sometimes with broad 'coathanger shoulders', but lighter in skeletal and muscle mass than mesomorphs, but also with low fat levels. Endomorphs tend to be rounder, wider hipped with high levels of bodyfat, especially round the middle, with a high waist to chest girth ratio. Although there are 3 main somatotypes, not everyone slots neatly into each category. Very often, individuals can be a mixture of 2 types. For example a slim athlete or endurance athlete may be a mixture of mesomorph-ectomorph and a female shotputter would be classed as a mesomorphic endomorph! The mesomorphic athletes tend to have a higher percentage of white fibred muscle whereas the endurance or ectomorphic athlete has a higher percentage of endurance or red fibred muscle. Obviously for the bodybuilding athlete, he is more likely to succeed with the mesomorph type physique.

2) Fibre Type As we have discussed in earlier chapters the training principles we use tends to use the white muscle fibres. As you will remember, we split these fibres into white glycolytic and white oxidative, but if we consider these just as a white fibre group now.

192

These are the fibres that we need a high percentage of in our bodies to successfully gain the muscle we need in bodybuilding. In order to test whether you have a genetic predisposition to gain, you can test your fibre type as follows. There are 3 variations to this test: One by Fred Hatfield, one by Charles Poliquin and another by Pipes. To make things easier and the results more well rounded we can use an amalgamation of all 3 tests. Now we need to look at upper and lower body. We need to select one exercise for overall lower body and one for upper body. As a lower body exercise, I would suggest squat for an experienced lifter, or leg press for inexperienced. Don't select leg extensions as I wouldn't suggest going for one rep maximums on this exercise due to too much stress on the cruciate ligaments. For the upper body, a barbell shoulder or chest press movement could be used. As there could be a comparison done with the pulling movements, you could include this too. Each rep must be performed strictly with a pause after each part of the movement, so momentum is taken out. After performing your warm ups carefully, you need to perform a one rep maximum on each of the exercises. Have a good, reliable spotter there if you can! This as you might guess is the maximum weight you can lift for one repetition. After resting 5 minutes, you then select 80% of this weight and then perform as many reps as you can with this weight, strictly. The results are interpreted in the table as follows:

MUSCLE FIBRE TESTING

NUMBER REPS PERFORMED AT 80% 1RM	MUSCLE FIBRE TYPE
LESS THAN 7 REPS	MOSTLY WHITE FAST TWITCH
7-10 REPS	MIXED FIBRE TYPE
GREATER THAN 10 REPS	MOSTLY RED SLOW TWITCH FIBRE

As you can see from the table, the top 2 categories which tend to suggest you have a higher percentage of white fibre in the muscle are the ideal categories you want to fall into to be more likely to build muscle strength and size. If you achieve more than 10 reps of your 80% 1 RM, then you are more likely to succeed in the endurance type sport arena. Sometimes, there can be variations in upper and lower body results. Some people tend to have higher red fibre percentage in their legs than upper body, having more trouble gaining in this area. In America, this sort of testing is done in collegiate sports to determine which sport or indeed which position would be best suited for each individual (eg in American Football) The main problem with this test is that it is rather nonspecific and only tests the muscle group being used in that exercise.

3) GENETIC MUTATED GENES:

Myostatin is a protein released by the muscle which inhibits the activation of satellite cells. These are the cells that allow the muscle to differentiate and grow. In other words, myostatin limits muscle growth. It has been noted in some animals and also used in breeding, that some animals with a mutated myostatin gene, that switches the myostatin receptors off, can put on 30% or more muscle than other breeds even when they are just standing around! This is clearly observed in Belgian Blue cattle (see previous picture). It has also been observed in humans. There are 2 groups of this mutated gene (homozygous and heterozygous), and can be detected from infancy in children that have an excessive amount of muscle for their age. It is likely that a fair percentage of top Professional Bodybuilders have this or a combination of these mutations. In my personal experience, working with top professionals, having trained with and treated a number of them, that they do not always train correctly or intensely. Many of them overtrain , sometimes twice daily, use volume training and do not hit maximum intensity, yet they still gain more muscle than your average bodybuilder who may train harder. However, I remember Dorian Yates once telling another top bodybuilder who was a genetic freak, 'You will never be Mr Olympia, unless you put my head on your shoulders!!'. He meant that unless he had Dorian's mindset, he would never make the most out of his superior genetics. So even the Myostain Mutated Bodybuilders would benefit even more if they trained properly!!

ACTN-3 Gene

Just recently this ACTN-3 Gene has been found in strength athletes, and especially sprinters. It allows the muscle to generate force very quickly in Glycolytic (Type 2X) white muscle fibres. When these athletes are subject to fast explosive training methods, their force development rate (RFD) comes on in leaps and bounds performance wise. We have known for a number of years that muscle fibre type has a strong bearing on the ability to generate force quickly. These type 2X or glycolytic muscle fibres contract much more quickly than other fibres and also are more involved in hypertrophy and strength than any other white fibres. The way we can apply this to our training in bodybuilding is to generate as much force as quickly as possible on the concentic or positive movement of an exercise. In other words, you are trying to move that weight as quickly as you can. Even

195

though the heavy weight still only moves slowly, the fact that your effort to move it quickly is what counts. Maximum force recruitment in these fibres leads to increased tension in the muscle meaning increased physiological adaptation, protein synthesis and therefore growth potential. It also means maximum motor unit recruitment meaning more muscle fibres are involved in this way.

The athlete that is blessed with higher ACTN-3 potential can improve his type 2X fibres in this way to a greater degree than someone who is not.

Although these gene mutated athletes may be gifted in this way, unless they apply correct training protocols, nutrition, rest etc., they will not achieve their full potential. You can only work with what you were born with, but its how you work with it that determines whether you reach your maximum potential. Even an average athlete can achieve phenomenal results if he or she applies these principles correctly and I am convinced that many athletes with the right mindset can overtake even athletes who are far more gifted genetically.

CHAPTER 11   ERGOGENIC AIDS: SUMMARY

Natural Ergogenics

Creatine: Either using monohydrate or ethyl ester versions requires no loading and up to 5-10 g per day can be used. Contrary to popular opinion there has been no long term kidney damage reported for dosages in this range. Always take with plenty of water for best results.

Testosterone Boosters: After numerous peer reviewed studies, up to date, only Vitamin D3 and zinc appreciably raise natural testosterone levels.
Growth Hormone Boosters: Good sleep patterns are essential, as well as rest from intense exercise. ProArgi 9+ produces a natural increase in GHRF when taken in 10g dosages just before retiring. Other supplements currently do not stack up to rigorous scientific scrutiny.

Berberine: Berberine can be used to improve insulin sensitivity and to control blood sugar levels. It is useful to take on high carb days as it helps insulin drive sugars from the blood into the cells and therefore is less likely for sugars to be laid down as bodyfat.

Unnatural Ergogenics:

Although I like to advise people against the use of exogenous testosterone and Growth Hormone, we have to accept that this practice goes on. I would rather guide people to do this under medical supervision and with the correct advice to minimise long term health implications than for them to fall under the auspices of some inscrutable 'so called guru'!!

Look out for signs of:

1)   Increased red blood cell count and Homocysteine levels
2)   Increased Blood Pressure
3)   Increased Fluid retention. (Swollen feet and ankles)

4) Numbness in the palm and aching in the wrist.
5) Check your blood sugar levels if using GH

Make sure you use the following supplements: Solgar's Homocysteine Modulator (or Trimethylglycine), Serrapeptase, Nattokinase, Enteric Coated Aspirin 75mg.

GENETICS

Somatotype and Fibre type: In order for you to determine your fibre type, perform as many reps as possible at your 80% 1 RM for 3 exercises: Squat, push, pull. Consult the table to see where your fibre type lies. This does not unduly affect the type of training you need to do to gain, as it is always mainly targeting the white fibre zone with the correct time under tension. This table just gives you an indication of your potential achievable with the correct training.

Myostatin and ACTN-3 Genes   Scientists have discovered mutations of the Myostatin gene and the presence of ACTN-3 gene in athletes with a much greater potential for gaining muscle mass and power output naturally.

198

CHAPTER 12 :
HEALTHY   BODYBUILDING   FOR
THE OVER 50's

Having reached this milestone myself, I and many of my contemporaries are now faced with a dilemma! How can we maintain a level of muscle and fitness at this age when all our joints and tissues are crying out no!! Hopefully this chapter will give you some insight as to how to achieve this without causing further damage preventing you ageing disgracefully!!

Ageing

You've often heard the expression, 'Age is just a number'!! Well it is actually - 2 numbers! Everyone has a Chronological age, but they also have a Biological age. Very often these two numbers don't match! Due to a number of factors that accumulate over time, such as physiological, psychological and social, the biological age can be a higher number than the chronological age! Physiological ageing is down to 2 groups of factors:

    1)   GENETIC factors
    2)   DAMAGE RELATED factors.

1) GENETIC FACTORS

Altered DNA Gene Transcrition: In a nutshell this means the the ability for the DNA to transcribe genes is reduced as one gets older. This is variable in different individuals

Telomere Shortening: The Telomere protects the ends of the chromosomes, but with every cell division they shorten. The length of the Telomere dictates how many times that particular cell can divide in a lifetime.

Decreased GH/ IGF-1 Signalling pathway: When GH signals more IGF-1 to be produced in the liver and cells, it then tells the cells to increase in protein synthesis, thereby repairing the cellular structures. As we age, this signalling process is reduced, resulting in less protein synthesis for cellular repair.

In the past, it was thought that these 3 main genetic factors causing ageing couldn't be altered through lifestyle choices. This doesn't, however seem to be the case. Just recently, Dr Elisabeth Blackburn won a Nobel Prize for her studies on Telomeres. Her book is called 'The Telomere Effect'. She described how you could affect your Telomere lifespan by regulating your sleep, exercise and nutrition patterns.

2) DAMAGE RELATED FACTORS:

By damage here, we are referring to direct DNA oxidative damage and Free-Radical damage to cells. As we have mentioned before, there are 2 pathways of oxidation to the body, one is 'clean' producing little or no damage to cells and one is 'dirty' producing damaging free radicals that act like 'shrapnel' to the cells. As also mentioned in the nutrition chapter, we recommend the use of antioxidants in food and supplement form to 'mop up' these damaging free radicals. There are various forms of oxidative damage done by different chemicals, so we need more than one antioxidant to deal with these. The main 4 antioxidants that work synergistically together are: Vitamin C, Selenium, Vitamin E , and Co-Enzyme Q10. These can massively help the cells to rejuvenate and also help to prevent abnormal cell mutations ie cancer cells developing.

Connective Tissues: Another problem with ageing is the loss of elastin connective tissue in structures like skin, tendons and ligaments. Collagen is also lost, reducing tensile strength of these structures. The elasticity of structures is so important for integrity of tissues. When this problem occurs in skin, it begins to sag, even under the sustained pressure of gravity. Cellular cross links also occur within tissues, making them much stiffer. Stiffness in these tissues also affects and damages vascular structures within the structure and therefore reduces blood and oxygen supply to the area.

So we can show that with the ageing process, although we may ultimately lose the war, we can win many battles along the way to delay the process and improve the quality of life! It's all about the correct balance of nutrition, exercise and rest. As we get chronologically older, we do have to reassess our type of exercise, the way we perform it, our scheduling, our nutrition and our rest patterns. As part of our exercise pattern, we need to look at our flexibility and pliability of our tissues. We need to include specific stretches for each muscle group regularly in our program. As a physiotherapist, I recommend static stretching. There are examples of this on the DVD. As you will see, as you breath out, you allow the stretch to occur slowly over a 30 second period. This allows stretch reflexes designed to protect the muscle and tendon to slowly ease down and allow the tissues to payout. NEVER stretch ballistically, bouncing at the end range!

With regard to aerobic/anaerobic training for the older athlete, if you want longevity of function and preservation of joint integrity, avoid ballistic exercises involving running and jumping. ie vigorous cross-fit , plyometrics and circuit training. All of these will give you a great overall fitness, but eventually at a cost! Train each facet of fitness separately, rather than trying to kill many birds with one stone as it were. Instead, for aerobic training, use nonballistic exercise machines such as a stationary bike, rowing machine, stepper or crosstrainer. Rather than doing long, drawn out aerobic sessions of 30 minutes plus which inhibits the anabolic response, use a short, sharp, intense loaded aerobic regime, using short, intense intervals, with little rest between, but that lasts less than 15 minutes. Training TABATA style, 3 times weekly massively improves your oxygen uptake, capillary density in muscles and lactate systems. It also helps to preserve muscle mass. In addition to this, long walks of submaximal intensity (30 mins or so) will help fat burning to boost metabolism.

With regard to sleep patterns, it has been shown that individuals getting 6-8 hours sleep at night drastically increase their life expectancy. Establishing a regular sleep pattern is of paramount importance with regard to recovery from exercise.

Although nutrition has been adequately covered in previous chapters, it must be emphasised that with regard to your micronutrition and the taking of antioxidants, to make sure you take them during the day before your workout and not straight away afterwards, as this can interfere with anabolic signalling after a workout. Although the ideal time to train regarding body rhythms is from 2 to 7 pm, some people have to train in the mornings. I would leave it 2-3 hours after then before taking any antioxidants of decent strength.

MICROBIOME

Recent scientific studies have uncovered a fascinating ecosystem within each of us called the MICROBIOME. This complex network of bacteria, fungi and microflora reside primarily in the gut and impact the health of virtually every system in the human body .The microbiome accounts for 90% of your cells in your body. Whilst the microbes living in your body are essential for your survival, imbalances in these can lead to all manner of health issues, some being the most chronic health issues of our time, like auti-immune diseases, MS, obesity, diabetes, asthma, rheumatism, cancer. Recent research also point towards our emotional and mental health being influenced by how well balanced our microbiome is!
Its interesting to note that all the billions of microbe cells that are contained within our bodies and are a part of us don't contain any of our DNA! Yet as we get older and our microbiome diminishes, then so can our immune system, recovery system and overall health. If we don't replenish this, it can have a serious effect on our ageing rate! So the 90% of your cells without your DNA are a massive help to the 10% of your cells WITH your DNA!! Very often, pollution in our atmosphere, chemicals in our environment, processed foods can all cause toxicity to our microbiome, causing an imbalance between the good and bad bacteria/microbes. Our friendly gut bacteria can be killed off in their millions!.The great thing about our microbiome system is that it is accessible and it can be modified. Three quarters of this system lives in your intestines. As we get older, we can top up our friendly microbes by adding PREBIOTICS and PROBIOTICS to our diets.

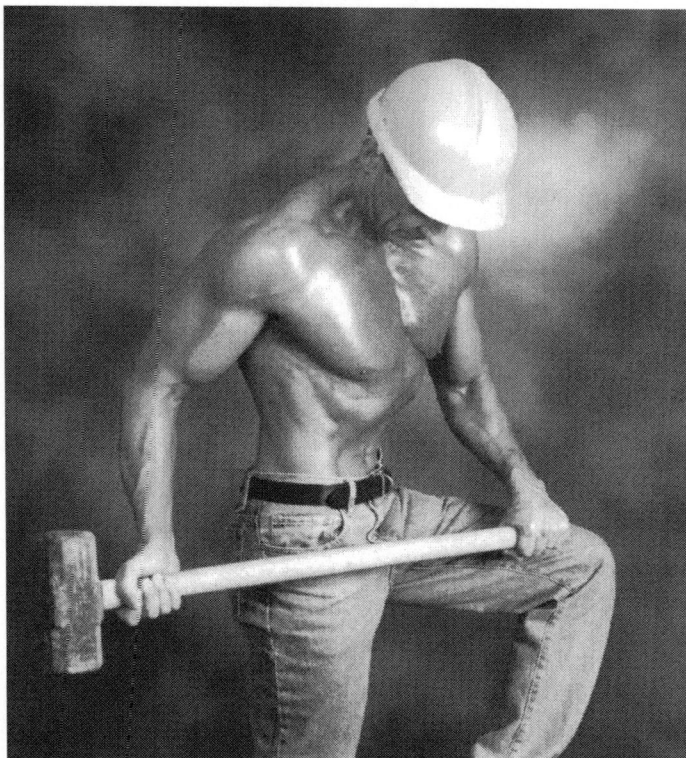

John Wardley: Came to me for advice on starting training at the age of 45 and achieved this amazing shape when he was 60!

PREBIOTICS:

Prebiotics are defined as nondigestible food fibres that can be utilised by probiotics. They are selectively utilised in the gut to increase friendly bacteria numbers. They aid digestion and enhance the production of valuable vitamins. They promote the growth of friendly bacteria without feeding the 'bad ' types. There is a group of polysaccharides known as Galactooligosaccharides (GOS) that form the most advanced Prebiotics. These are nutrient fibres. The main source of prebiotics in foods is the INULIN found in Jerusalem artichokes, garlic, asparagus and leeks. The only problem it is in such poor quantities that you would have to consume masses of these food to really benefit fully. Whilst we recommend these foods in your diet, we also recommend you supplement with INULIN or GOS as well. Whilst all prebiotics are fibre, not all fibres are prebiotics! The common forms of dietary fibre present in the majority of plant based foods and grains are less selectively fermented by the bacteria in the gut and lack some of the health benefits demonstrated by prebiotics. However, they are still of benefit to our health and their consumption is to be encouraged as they help maintain regular toilet habits as well as promoting the health of the gut itself.

One of the prebiotic products we recommend is BIMUNO. This contains the most advanced prebiotic GOS (Galactooligosaccharide). It is in the form of a satchet you mix in your fruit juice as is flavorless.

PROBIOTICS

Probiotics are live, active bacteria such as bifidobacteria and lactobacilli that are exogenous and enter the gut by the ingesting of foods and supplements. There are many 1000's of strains of bacteria, but not all of these are friendly to our systems. The ingestion of 'bad' bacteria such as Heliobactor Pylori can cause ulcers and damage to the intestines. There are about 5-10 strains of 'friendly' bacteria that the gut needs for essential health. These tend to include the lactobacilli and the bifidobacteria. A good probiotic supplement we recommend is by Solgar and is the 40+ Advanced Acidophilus.

Modifications to the Resistance Program for the Over 50's

As we have seen in previous chapters, correct periodisation is necessary for any age of strength athlete to achieve their potential, but especially for the older strength athlete. Microtear damage and microlesions in the muscles can lead to further damage, resulting in a breakdown of tissue which overides that of anabolic repair. This can lead to an inefficiency of the muscle contraction, inhibition of the neuromuscular system, which then leads to injury. As we get older, the GH signalling system from resistance training is much reduced. In fact GH and IGF-1 levels decline at an exponential rate from aged 40. In order to try to kick start this system again, we can change our style of training. It has been shown that isoforms of IGF-1 directly formed in the muscle can be dramatically increased when we switch to slow eccentric training. Eccentric training should now take precedence over glycolytic training. The main localised isoform produced is MGF. (mechano growth factor). FGF (fibroblastic growth factor) is also stimulated to help improve the integrity of ligaments and tendons when put under this more sustained loading.

I would recommend the following program as a modified program from that set out earlier in this book:
WEEK 1:   ECCENTRIC
WEEK 2:   OXIDATIVE (15 rep working set)
WEEK 3:   GLYCOLYTIC
WEEK 4:   ECCENTRIC
Repeat this cycle one more time, then take a full week off resistance training and just do aerobics and fat burning. Do not for one minute think you will lose muscle mass by taking 1 week off. If anything, you will come back STRONGER !!
When doing the Oxidative week, you have the option of increasing reps to a maximum of 15, giving a time under tension of 75 secs, or just increase your slow negative time under tension from 1minute (6 slow reps) to 1 and half minutes (9

205

slow reps). The glycolytic set should only last for 30 secs of sustained tension (6 to 8 reps).

To Press or Not to Press?

Bodybuilders from a young age are indoctrinated with a common policy. You MUST press and you must do compound movements! So they get on the conveyor belt of multiple bench pressing, chest pressing at multiple angles, shoulder pressing, sometimes even (dare I say it) behind the neck pressing. As a Physio over many years, I have seen the results of this policy manifest in terms of fixed postural tension, rotator cuff lesions, shoulder and elbow arthritis etc. I would therefore recommend, even the younger athlete to reduce volume and number of pressing movements. I would suggest only one compound pressing movement for chest and only one pressing movement for shoulders, followed by more isolation movements. For the older over 50's bodybuilder, I would suggest NO PRESSING AT ALL!! If you want to help preserve your joint spaces, articular cartilage and help your rotator cuff, then isolate only!

TYPICAL CHEST PROGRAM

INCLINE FLYES (dumbells)

STANDING PULLEY CABLE FLYES (from high position to low)

PEC DECK INNER RANGE

Perform these exercises in strict form, with pauses at each end of a full range of movement. Incline bench should only be set at an angle no more than 30 degrees.

Before you start, always warm-up the rotator cuff and scapular stabilisers with some pulley or dumbbell lateral rotation work to activate these muscles. When you start any flying movement, you need to 'set up your base' as it where, activating your lats and retractors statically to 'lock in' your scapulae and create a strong base to drive from and also preventing overprotraction of the shoulders. **Check out the exercises on the DVD**

TYPICAL SHOULDER PROGRAM

FRONT RAISE

LATERAL RAISE (2 angles)

SHRUGS

Again, start with your rotator cuff lateral rotation exercises, before you start the first exercise. Front raise can be done using dumbbells or a 'D' bar. It is safer to use a midposition grip, getting a hold at a 90 degree position. Do not raise too high or subacromial compression can be a problem. Do not 'swing', but use a back-rest to stop this happening. Always control the descent even when you aren't doing deliberate eccentric work. Pause at each end of the range to create more tension within the muscle. This will strongly activate your anterior deltoid.

Laterals should be done at 2 angles, as 2 separate exercises. The first angle is done by leaning your chest against an incline bench, just offset from the vertical. Lift your arms out with your palms slightly pronated. Try to get a strong hold momentarily at 90 deg, before controlling the descent. Keep a tension on at the bottom, not completely relaxing the deltoid before you rise again. After your warm-ups and working set for this exercise, reset the bench angle so it is at 45 deg. Then, leaning against this, perform the lateral movement again. This angle is higher than a completely bent over position, but it takes even more off the anterior delt and puts the tension on the rear/lateral heads. It is a kind of hybrid movement. As you work your retractors (Rhomboids and middle traps) strongly during your back workouts, we don't want to do a purely 'bent-over' movement and overlap these muscle groups. Then, following this, traps, already partially worked can be worked to failure.

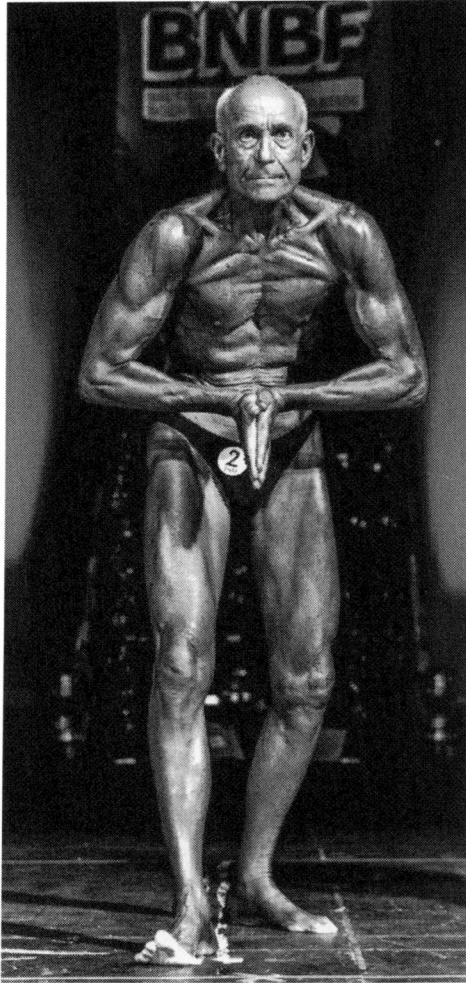

Pete Elmes: A most inspirational man! Despite having a serious life threatening cancer and whilst undergoing chemotherapy, he achieved this condition, qualifying for the BNBF British Finals in the Over 70's category. I am proud to know and train him!

Do not be misled into thinking that your deltoids cannot reach or maintain maximum potential without pressing. Believe me, they can and can even improve without compromising your chance of injury and longevity, training at maximum intensity for as long as you can!

Preventative Therapy (Prophylactic Treatment):

As I have already mentioned, it is very important for any athlete, and especially the older athlete to undergo a strict stretching protocol both daily and prior to heavy exercise. The DVD associated with this book goes through some important stretches and how to perform them. In short, each stretch should be held for 30 secs to relax the stretch reflexes and allow the muscle fibres to pay out. During the 30secs, breathing out when you progress the stretch is important and adds to the relaxation and lengthening effect.

Linked with this, it is important to maintain the integrity and flexibility of the fascia which covers and intersperses the muscle. As we have previously discussed, the fascia has strong correlation with muscle function. If it is damaged or adhesed, then maximal muscle contraction is inhibited. A dropping off of performance or dysfunction of a particular movement will be noticed. This is a good time to get this problem fixed. As physiotherapists we are very 'Hands on' and consider regular treatment of the fascia to be of prime concern to the athlete who wants to maximise his potential. Techniques such as Fascial Release, Active release and Acupuncture are done to release the fascia and improve blood flow to the muscles. Some techniques are demonstrated on the DVD. Many of the top Professional Bodybuilders such as Ronnie Coleman in his prime regularly used therapists trained in these fields. We have many top strength athletes having regular check ups of the soft tissues in our clinic. I used to regularly make the trip down to Dorian's house to train with him and treat him afterwards. He saw the importance of the link between regular physio and performance.

Associated with this fascial tension is postural tension which can build up over a number of months and can be a major problem!

Once the fascia tightens and shortens, it can severely affect posture. If this process is allowed to continue, then reflex actions associated with joints can cause a sensitisation of the area. This particularly happens with the spine. Due to mechanoreceptors in the facet joints of the vertebrae, a sensitive reflex action can be set up, which can easily cause muscle spasm and a 'locking' of this area of the spine. Many patients report an innocuous action which seems to cause this, such as bending to pick up a drawing pin or other light object and the whole system of overprotection fires up! This can severely restrict function and is horrendously painful. We constantly have to council patients that the innocuous act of picking up a light object was simply 'the straw that broke the camels back', meaning the final instigation of the spasm set up by a long term build up of postural tension! They DO NOT as some other therapists have told them have a 'weak back', or a 'weak core'. It always makes me chuckle when one of our bodybuilder or powerlifting patients comes in and reports they have a weak core!! I tell them, if you have a 'weak core', then how is it you can squat with over 400Ilbs? That seems to reassure them! It could be that they have a 'poor core endurance', but certainly not a weak one! However, this is not the initial issue. The first priority is to free off the locked spinal segments through manipulation and acupuncture, followed by release of all the soft-tissues. This is repeated until we 'reset' their mechanoreceptors. Then the whole system will restabilise and their function and power will return. We then attempt to reeducate their thinking both in their need to periodise their training better and to get monthly, bimonthly or trimonthly checkups to maintain their function according to their individual requirements.

RED LIGHT THERAPY

In recent years, a Harvard Professor, Michael Hamblin has done over 300 studies irradiating patients with many different wavelengths of Infra-Red and Visible red concentrated light sources. He found that out of the whole spectrum of Infra-Red and Red light, there were 2 very distinct slices of wavelengths that massively increased mitochondrial activities in cells. This means the metabolism of the cellular activity was drastically increased. This quickly steps up the healing potential of damaged tissues. These 2 wavelengths were 660nm (Infra-red) and 850 nm (visible red). The 660nm wavelength penetrated very deep into the deeper soft-tissues, but not through bone. The 850nm penetrated to dermis depth in skin. Therefore, by taking these 2 wavelengths and incorporating them into a large surface area lamp, with many LED's emitting these 2 wavelengths, a large area of the body could be treated at once.

Benefits of Red Light Therapy

It is through this hike in cellular metabolism that Red Light Therapy has been shown to aid in muscular recovery, both after intense training and also following injury.

It has also been proven to improve skin tone, clarity and texture, diminishing age-spots and improving fine lines and wrinkles Having used it at our clinic for the last 2 years, I have noticed a number of patients for whom their scars and blemishes have reduced or disappeared! They also notice an improvement in energy levels, reduction in joint pain and enhanced cognitive function. The only draw back is the need for regular treatment on a daily basis to get the most out of the treatment. I tend to recommend intense courses when time allows, as the effects do diminish when usage ceases. It also needs to be allied to a good nutritional program and I usually advise people to think of it as another anti-ageing tool to be used when they can.

Andropause

Simply put, as the male ages, beyond late 40's, the production of testosterone by the pituitary gland severely diminishes. Any man with a Total Testosterone level of 10nmol/litre or less is considered to be in Andropause if this level stays the same or lower over a 6 month period. This, allied to below normal levels of FSH (Follicle stimulating hormone) and LH (luteinising Hormone) is further evidence of Andropause. If we now look at the diagram headed MALE TESTICULAR AXIS we can see how the brain works through a series of hormonal stimuli to produce the testosterone. The area of the brain called the Hypothalamus, stimulates the pituitary gland to produce FSH and LH using the Gonadotrophin Releasing Hormone (GRH). These in enough quantities ie in a +ve state tell the testes to produce testosterone via the Leydig cells and sperm via the sertoli cells. As you can see, there is a negative feedback mechanism also involved. If a person takes too much outside (exogenous) testosterone then over production of DHT and Oestrogen as the testosterone aromatises then causes the pituitary gland and hypothalamus to produce less gonadotrophins or less GRH, FSH and LH. This results in less natural (endogenous) testosterone production. This shuts down the whole axis if allowed to continue for too long. In severe cases, the younger athlete can even be rendered sterile! In the older athlete, whether there is an exogenous supply of testosterone or not, there will slowly be a diminishing of GRH as the axis begins to diminish.

Another hormone called SHBG (sex hormone binding Globulin) pulls usable testosterone from the blood and binds it up so it cannot activate receptor sites in cells. The free testosterone or usable testosterone is in the plasma of the blood and can attach to receptor sites to pass its message onto the cells. This level of free testosterone to bound can also be affect as we get older, resulting in less free testosterone getting through to the cells.

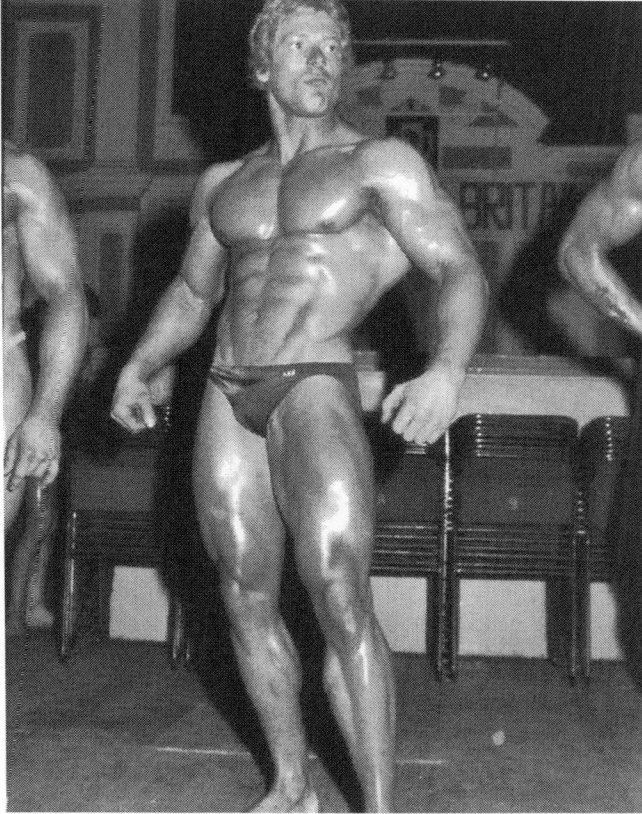

Gordon Pasquill: This photo of Gordon taken in his '20s was my first local bodybuilding hero! He is the only bodybuilder to win all the classes from junior to senior over 50's at the NABBA Mr UK competitions. I was privileged to prep him for his over 50's titles.

MALE TESTICULAR AXIS

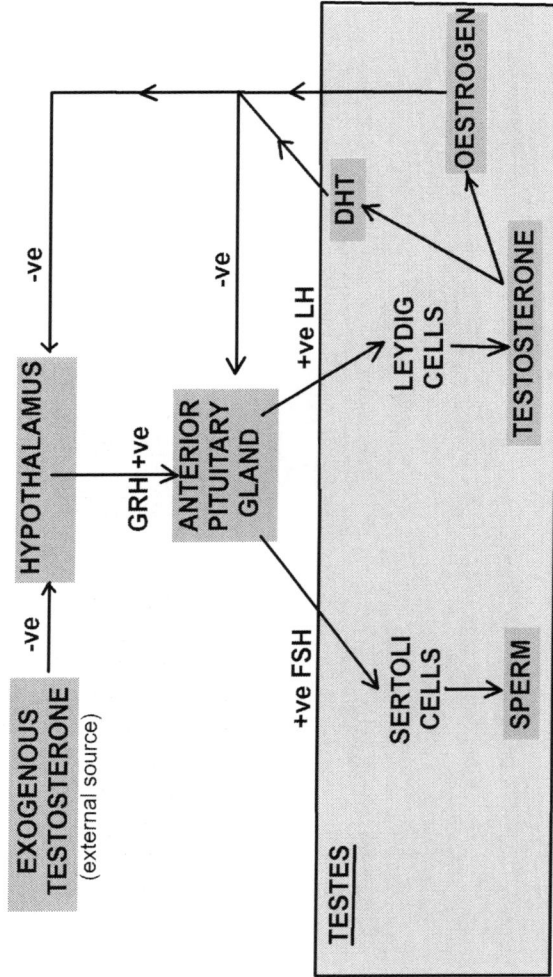

EXOGENOUS TESTOSTERONE
(external source)

-ve

HYPOTHALAMUS

-ve

GRH +ve

ANTERIOR PITUITARY GLAND

-ve

+ve FSH

+ve LH

DHT

OESTROGEN

LEYDIG CELLS

TESTOSTERONE

SERTOLI CELLS

SPERM

TESTES

FSH - Follicle Stimulating Hormone   LH - Luteinising Hormone   GRH - Gonadotropin Releasing Hormone

214

Symptoms of Andropause

Low Libido
Depression
Low energy levels
Erectile Dysfunction
Increased Bodyfat levels
Increased Irritability
Cardiovascular problems
Osteoporosis

Treatment

As we spoke about in the younger athlete, if we need to increase testosterone, we need to do Intense Resistance Exercise.

The taking of supplements Zinc and Vitamin D3 can also help to keep the Testicular Axis viable.

However, as you get into your 50's. this form of treatment becomes less effective. If after trying the above for 6 months and you still have low Testosterone, FSH and LH levels, then I would refer the patient to see his GP with a view to seeing an endocrinologist. The endocrinologist may then try to re-establish his GRH with treatment. If this proved unsuccessful, then they would use HRT (Hormone Replacement Therapy). The sad state of affairs in the UK is that Andropause (unlike Menopause) for women is not widely recognised even by some endocrinologists. I always tell the patients I advise to get on their 'soapbox' about it and kick up a fuss, as this is a REAL condition which can have severe repercussions on biological ageing and health if not addressed. It sometimes appears that whether through cost savings or ignorance that older people are left to age disgracefully! It is surely all about 'quality of life' and treating Andropause just symptomatically i.e. Antidepressants, Viagra etc. is just not good enough!

FEMALE OVARIAN AXIS

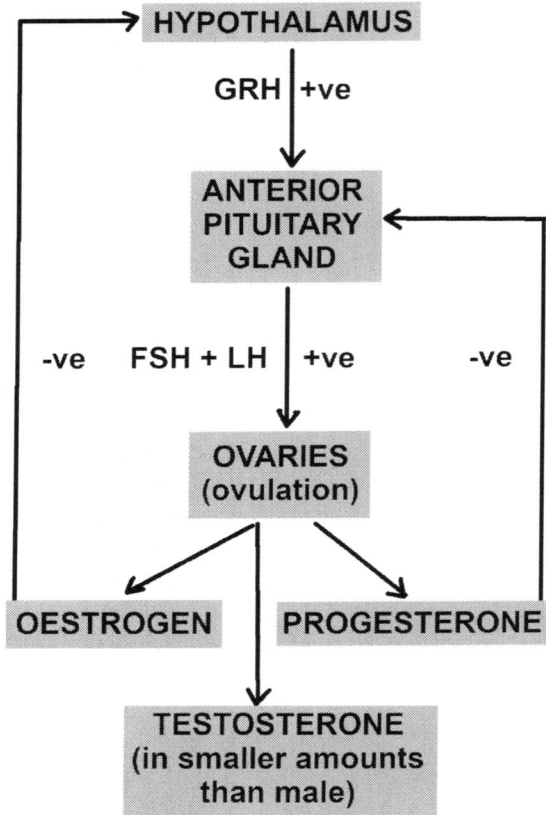

HYPOTHALAMUS

GRH | +ve

ANTERIOR
PITUITARY
GLAND

-ve   FSH + LH | +ve   -ve

OVARIES
(ovulation)

OESTROGEN   PROGESTERONE

TESTOSTERONE
(in smaller amounts
than male)

Female Ovarian Axis

As you can see from the DIAGRAM, it is a similar system that fuels the female ovarian axis, except the main concern here is the maintenance of the female characteristics that produce ovulation for procreation. However, it must be noted that the female does in fact produce a small degree of useable testosterone and maintenance of this is also important. Very often, when women are treated for Menopause, they are usually given an oestogen or combination oestogen/progesterone hormone replacement, but they are very rarely given a testosterone replacement. During menopause, if testosterones diminish as well, then loss of bone and muscle mass can occur. Female hormone replacements go a long way to benefitting the bone loss, but also cause more water and fat retention and don't do enough to maintain muscle mass. There is a good hormone precursor called Tibolone which can be used as an alternative as it converts to oestrogen, progesterone and androgen hormones in the body with less risk of breast cancer. The use of a Testosterone Gel like Tostran could also be used to boost female androgens. It can go a long way to help female energy levels, libido, muscle mass and training potential. The dosage has to be carefully managed to prevent masculisation effects, but mostly it can be well managed.

SARMS

Recently there are a new group of substances under analysis. These actually modify the receptor sites for testosterone Recent studies have shown one particular substance called Ostarine for combatting Andropause in men and also for use with women also. It was under investigation initially to try to prevent osteoporosis. The only problem with SARMS is that they are sold along with many other banned substances. They are marketed in such a way as to convince the athlete they will test negative for controlled substances. More research needs to be done to make sure these are effective enough to be used in an Andropause situation.

217

HRT THERAPY FOR MEN

Once the endocrinologist or GP has fully investigated the Testicular Axis and found that treatment for the pituitary gland to rejuvenate the axis has not been successful, then HRT should be administered. This will reduce all the symptoms described earlier for Andropause. It will also prevent the older man from suffering SARCOPENIA or severe muscle loss as a result of very low androgen levels. This is a condition that mainly affects the older man, especially the older man who doesn't do any resistance training. It can start from as early as 40 years, but especially in his 50's, the man who does not do resistance training will lose muscle exponentially, usually putting fat on as well as the turnover metabolically in the muscle is severely affected. The Hormones administered in HRT must be administered under medical control. It would be unwise to try to administer these drugs yourself without the correct advice. It is a very complex system and as is common with the hormone system, small changes don't always manifest straight away, but very much in a timed-delay fashion. Homeostasis of the bodies hormone system sometimes takes years to get right with Hormone therapy, so patience is a virtue. Overdosing for long periods could severely damage your health and the main reason you are doing it in the first place. Whilst normal levels of Testosterone benefits the cardiovascular system, too large a dose for extended periods could have life threatening results!

Whilst undergoing HRT therapy with Testosterone, it is important to recognise the main blood parameters that have to be kept under control. As Homocysteine levels rise, it is important to check they are within safe parameters. Too high a level over a period of time can lead to a hardening of the arteries and a risk of life threatening thrombus or embolus formation. Another main blood factor to be aware of is rises in the level of Red Blood cells. Testosterone increases the body's production of red blood cells. This in moderation is a good thing as it helps prevent anaemia and supplies the tissues with adequate oxygen. However, if levels rise too much, then the viscosity of the blood can get to a level where the blood thickens and deoxygenates the tissues as the red cells clump. This can lead to thrombus formation and can be life threatening.

The main blood tests to undergo every few months whilst on HRT are:

Homocysteine Levels

FBC (full blood count) which incorporates Haematocrit (the level of cells versus fluid in the blood) and red blood cell count.

Testosterone Levels

PSA levels (To be dealt with later in this chapter)

Supplements:

I thoroughly recommend the following supplements to safeguard you in this regard. Serrapeptase, a proteolytic enzyme which helps to break down protein debris in the body. Taken early morning, before breakfast on an empty stomach. Also, along with this, Nattokinase, an enzyme which helps the body break down the fibrin part of any clot formation. Daily dosage of 75mg Enteric Aspirin can also be a lifesaver as this helps to keep the blood 'slippery' and flowing. It has also been shown to help guard against colonic cancer. Being enteric coated helps protect it from irritating the stomach.

If the levels of Haematocrit and Red blood cell concentrations rise too high then obviously this can be dose dependant and adjustments in the HRT need to be made. If after this, levels are still dangerous, then the only option would be to undergo 'blood letting' by a phlebotomist. Another option is to have a course of 'Therapeutic Ultrasound' which when applied at the correct dosage to main arteries such as carotid or femoral can break down red blood cells to a safer range. Studies have shown that Naringin found in Grapefruits can also lower haematocrit. Half a grapefruit per day is enough to lower red blood cell count. TrimethylGlycine helps the body 'mop' up excessive levels of

Homocysteine. The best supplement I know in this regard is Solgar's Homocysteine Modulator.

Somatopause

Somatopause is the condition described when the own bodies Growth Hormone and Insulin Growth Factor production lowers to a level below that of normal for your age group and never recovers. This occurs as part of the biological ageing process. The area of the brain called the Hypothalamus produces a naturally occurring GHRH (Growth Hormone Releasing Hormone). This then tells the Pituitary Gland to produce more GH and IGF. (Growth Hormone and Insulin Growth Factors) IGF is then mainly formed from this response in the Liver and Isoforms of this are formed directly in tissues eg Muscle tissue. These then improve protein synthesis in connective tissues and muscles which stimulates fat metabolism also. Growth Hormone levels are at a maximum during childhood, slowly depleting in the late teens and 20's, dropping to 25% of this level by the time you reach your 40's and 50's.

Symptoms of Somatopause

Decreased Muscle mass (sarcopenia)
Increased Fat mass
Decreased energy levels
Loss of Elastin in skin ie more wrinkles and sagging skin
Loss of Bone Density ie osteopenia or osteoporosis
General lack of well being and libido
Increase in Total Cholesterol

Treatment

Intense resistance training and short intense aerobic/anaerobic exercise increases your bodies own growth hormone production.

Good quality sleep pattern of at least 7+ hours per night.

However, as we get older, our pulsatile releases of GH during the day and night get lower in intensity due to the less

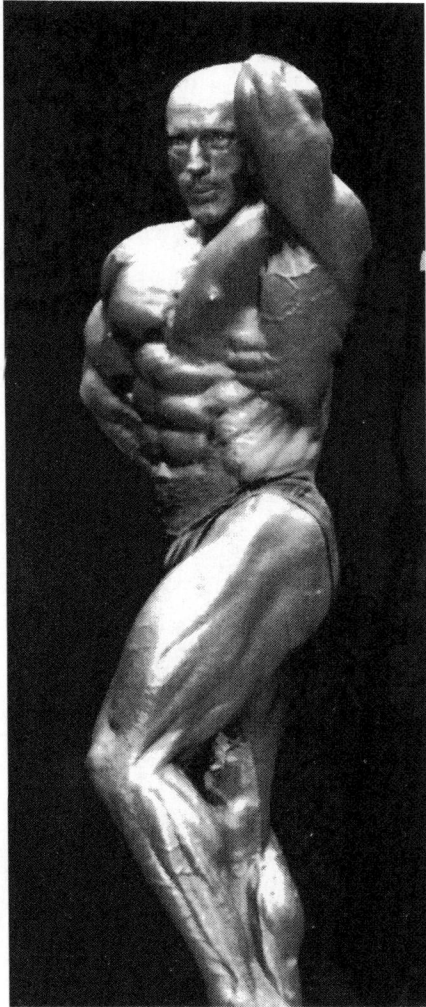

Dave Steele: A multiple British and Universe title winner in the Over 50's. A fantastic example of what can be achieved by the older bodybuilder!

stimulation from the hypothalamus. This is mainly due to the diminishing of the regulator hormone GHRF. In order to maximise this production, it has been shown that the amino-acid L-Arginine when taken at night in high enough quantities can be beneficial. However, L-Arginine is what is termed a blind amino acid, meaning when it enters the system it is not always directed where to go in a cellular sense. By taking it with an amino-acid rider to get it across the blood brain barrier, it can then influence the hypothalamus. As mentioned before, Synergy's ProArgi9 seems to have the formula which is most productive. Studies show that after 6 months, IGF-1 levels can be restored . It also has circulatory benefits through nitric -oxide stimulation on the endothelial cells of arteries, massively improving their efficiency and overall cardio-vascular health.

The formula Synergy use for their ProArgi9 contains the highest pharmaceutical grade of Arginine with a low glycemic natural glycoside from the plant 'stevia'. It also combines the arginine with Vitamin K,D3 and C which potentiate its response along with L-Citrulline which keeps the arginine active for longer in the body. This formula needs to be taken at least 2 hours after your last meal, and 15-30 minutes before retiring to bed. The dosage generally needs to be 10g or 2 satchets to get maximum growth hormone stimulation.

HRT for Somatopause

There are a number of Anti-aging clinics to be found in the USA. A lot of these provide people with private prescriptions of GH straight away. This is very expensive and for some illegitimate clinics it is a money making racket. Some of the more decent clinics will carefully study your test results before determining what you need. Very often, it is found, especially in the 50's that GH response is down for your age , purely because your GHRF is reduced. The GHRF can be sequenced and made in the lab. It is called Sermorelin. This is a synthetic version and replaces your GHRF produced by your Hypothalamus. It is therefore higher up the chain of production and encourages

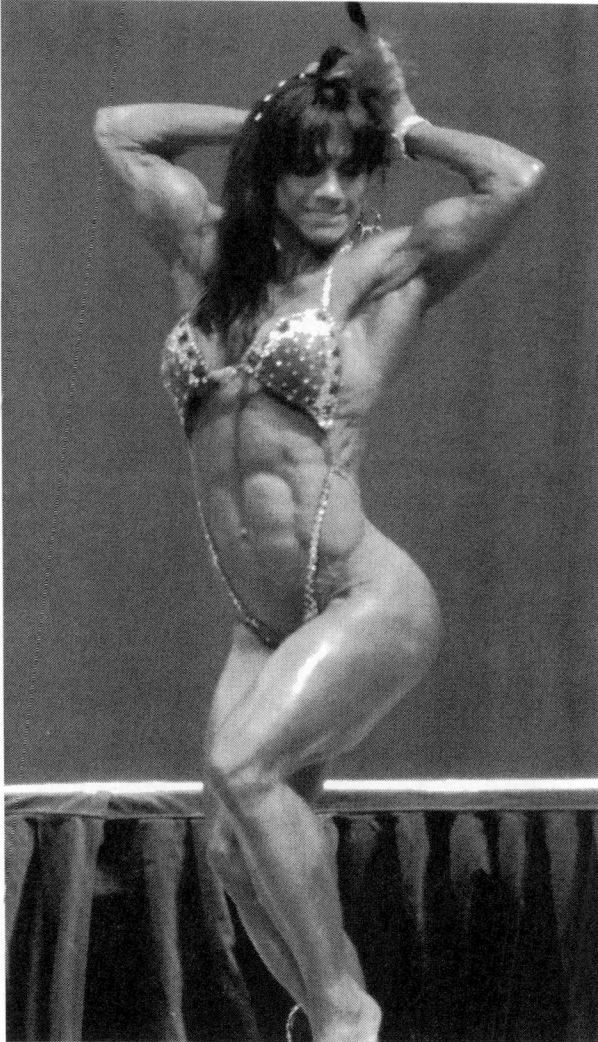

Cheryl Steele: Wife of Dave Steele and winner of 3 British Titles. She achieved this condition at age 58 when she was a grandmother!!

your body to produce more of its own GH and IGF. This is much better initially than just taking GH. If you took GH when your GHRF was trying to recover, it would shut it down completely. Using Sermorelin is a much safer alternative and causes less side effects. Although most clinics offering GH therapy only use small doses to mimic a younger persons GH response, some people have strong receptor affinity to a sudden increase. Although it is unlikely these recipients will get side effects on a par with bodybuilders who overdose, it is worth bearing in mind that long-term use needs to be carefully monitored. The main tests to keep an eye on for Somatopause HRT patients are : regular blood sugar checks, and 6 monthly tests for IGF-1 and IGF-BP3. As levels of GH rise and fall during the day and night, these fluctuations make it hard to access. IGF-1 levels are more stable and one only needs to fast overnight and do a morning sample for an accurate result. IGF-BP3 is the carrier for IGF-1 and is also a good indicator of Somatopause.

Normal level range for IGF-BP3 for male aged 50-60 should be : 3.4 to 6.9 mcg/ml. This figure is similar for females of this age.

Normal levels for IGF-1 for males (50 to 60): 51 to 194 ng/ml and for females: 45-173 ng/ml.

If your levels for both these fall below these levels for this age bracket, then you can consider yourself to be in Somatopause.

Haemodynamics

Yes, it's a bit of a mouthful isn't it! In short, it just means 'the dynamics of blood flow'. Blood flow around the body is dependant on so many factors such as the healthiness of the heart and blood vessels, the hormone systems that control it, the thickness of the blood and the pliabilty of the tissues it has to traverse through. Poor blood flow restricts the delivery of oxygen, nutrients and hormones to all areas of the body. It can severely impede protein synthesis in tissues, resulting in poor recovery, and poor transport of waste products away from tissues to the kidneys. This can cause back pressure, clogging up the system and further impeding nutrients delivery to tissues.

As we have already discussed, poor posture and tension can happen to anyone, but is even more prevalent and can build up over longer periods in older athletes. This situation needs to be addressed to prevent serious impeding of blood flow. It is even more imperative that the older bodybuilder have regular check ups of his soft and hard tissues. Regular physio check ups can cover all these areas.

POSTURE: Regular assessments every few months can detect any postural changes which can be corrected early and given the right program.

HARD TISSUES: By this I mean the joint structures. Spinal segments and other synovial joints can become tight and stiff due to incorrect posture and tension. This is corrected using manipulation techniques, mobilisation techniques, acupuncture. Regular releases of these hard tissues stops abnormal reflex action building up which alters posture and sensitises the stress response.

SOFT-TISSUES: Using fascial release and active release techniques, we can relieve the soft tissues of stress and tension. Then to help blood flow we can improve soft tissue pliabilty with stretch techniques, postural positioning and endurance work, along with acupuncture.

Regular sports massages in between the physio sessions is also recommended.

Supplements such as Proargi9+ and Niacin help nitric oxide production which has a direct effect on endothelial cells in blood vessels and helps improve haemodynamics.

CRAMP: Cramp in its many forms is more predominant in the older athlete. Sometimes it can be as a result of dehydration, but more often it is due to altered blood flow. Very often it can occur soon after intense resistance exercise very often in the

225

legs. The actin/myosin cross ridges which form the contractile element in muscles in action also form when at rest. Usually an 'action potential' is set up in the nerve muscle connection and the actin protein cannot release its hold! The muscle then cannot release the contraction and it quickly becomes 'ischaemic' shutting its own blood supply down. Relaxing this action potential can be done by restoring the calcium pump mechanism in the muscle back to normal, usually by taking calcium and magnesium in supplement form. If one adds Niacin to the mix, then this can quickly dilate the blood vessels, restoring circulation. It's a shame that the supplement 'crampex' was inadvertently taken off the market as its composite calcium, magnesium and niacin combination worked a treat for those people suffering from cramp, especially night cramps. Often Doctors prescribe quinine, but this is very liver toxic!

Cramps suffered by intense resistance trainers are not usually through electrolyte imbalance as can sometimes be a cause as they usually hydrate and mineralise their bodies with adequate nutrition.

The Prostate Gland

All men have a prostate, an apricot sized, muscular gland that produces some of the ingredients of semen. It sits just in front of the rectum and below the bladder. It surrounds the urethra, the tube that takes the urine from the bladder to the penis. It is vital for the proper function of the male reproductive system. It secretes a fluid that keeps the sperm alive while protecting them and the genetic code they carry. The prostate contracts during ejaculation and squirts its fluid into the urethra. The prostate contracts and closes off the opening between the bladder and urethra to stop urine mixing with the semen as it is forcibly pushed through. This prostatic fluid contains enzymes, zinc and citric acid. It helps the sperm to live as long as possible to allow fertilisation to occur. One of the enzymes produced is PSA (Prostate Specific Antigen). This helps the sperm thin down as it enters the vagina so it is more likely to reach the egg. To function properly, the Prostate needs testosterone and DHT (Dihydrotestosterone).

226

Benign Prostatic Hypertrophy

All men over age 50 suffer from this to varying degrees. DHT receptor sites in the prostate cause it to enlarge to varying degrees. BPH as it is known can be so slow growing that it causes only minimal symptoms. However, it can cause frequent and painful urination in more severe cases. In most cases this condition is benign and an elevated PSA level indicates an increase in metabolic processes in the prostate and needs to be monitored. If evidence of Prostate cancer is eliminated, then the drug of choice to reduce the size of the Prostate is <u>Finasteride</u>. This reduces the androgen DHT and prevents the Prostate enlarging, allowing better urine flow. The main side effects can be impotence and loss of libido, but in doses of 5mg daily, this isn't usually a problem. Because it blocks DHT receptor sites, it can also prevent or restore hair loss! BPH is usually diagnosed through rectal examination, ultrasound scan and PSA level checks. One of the natural supplements that has shown promise in helping BPH is <u>Saw Palmetto</u>. Results have only been good if the product is taken consistently for long periods i.e. 12 months or longer.

Prostate Cancer

Despite Prostate cancer being one of the most prevalent cancers in males, most BPH sufferers do not suffer from it. Very often, men with high PSA levels are quickly sent for a Prostate Biopsy, sometimes unnecessarily! This is a very invasive, painful procedure which involves going through the rectal wall to take a chunk out of the prostate for analysis. In fact, many tiny chunks are taken, leaving the patient open to infections, possible urinary incontinance and impotence due to damage to important nerves in the area! If there are no symptoms of possible CaProstate such as blood in urine, painful urination, decreased urine flow, then a PSA test is not an indicator to proceed with a Biopsy. Prostate cancer is normally very slow growing and most men die with prostate cancer, not from it. Although regular PSA tests can be useful to see what is going on over a period of time, it is a poor indicator to detect cancer. It certainly can't detect whether the cancer is slow or fast growing! Another factor to consider when undergoing PSA testing is the result may depend on what you did just prior to the test. For example, a man who cycles to the doctors to have a test will have a higher level than if he went by car! Testing of PSA should also not follow rectal examination, high intensity exercise or after sex. All these events can cause abnormal temporary rises in PSA leading to a false reading!

Other Screening Tests for Prostate Cancer

Unfortunately, on the NHS, other screening other than PSA and Prostate Biopsy is not available. However there are other effective tests which are non invasive which can be done.

PCA 3 Test: This is a new gene based test carried out on a urine sample. It is highly specific to prostate cancer and this gene is expressed in over 95% of prostate cancer cases. This is in contrast to PSA which can also be increased by BPH and Prosatatitis (Inflammation of the prostate). The PCA 3 test is not affected by these conditions. The PCA 3 test looks for the expression of genes found only in prostate cancer cells. Up to 100 times more PCA 3 is present in prostate cancer cells than non-cancerous cells. By analysing cells from the prostate found in the urine, the likelihood of having a prostate cancer can be determined.

Urine Exosome Gene Expression Assay : This test measures not just PCA 3, but also 2 other genes associated with high grade disease: ERG and SPDEF. The test combines these measures into a diagnostic score that could help determine if a Biopsy is necessary or not. One of its developers, Dr Michael Donovan reinforced that the goal was to limit the number of prostate cancer biopsies done which are costly, painful and prone to hospital acquired infections.

CHAPTER 12: HEALTHY BODYBUILDING FOR THE OVER 50's SUMMARY

1) Ageing has a chronological number and a biological number. Only the biological number can for a time be reduced.

2) Damage factors affecting the cells can be reduced by the taking of anti-oxidants both in food and supplement form. The 'big four' are selenium. vitamin C, vitamin E , and Co-Enzyme Q10.

3) Signalling factors for the release of GH (Growth hormone) and IGF-1 can be increased by taking Pro-Argi9+ It also releases Nitric-oxide which improves the health and circulatory supply by the arteries to improve oxygen supply to tissues.

4) Getting at least 7 hours of quality sleep per night also helps signalling pathways for GH and also helps repair the neural system and immune system.

5) Red light Therapy can be used to increase metabolism by increasing mitochondrial activity in cells so this helps their repair processes. It can help muscle repair at 850nm and skin blemishes and wrinkles at 660nm.

6) Physiotherapy: Regular check ups for posture, release of joint adhesions, active and fascial release techniques for soft tissues should be done to help maintain performance and prevent injury. Massage techniques can be done even more frequently to help maintain soft-tissue integrity.

7) Microbiome: In order to improve the micro-organisms living in our gut, we need to take extra strains of 'friendly bacteria' and fuel them with a Prebiotic. The 2 supplements we recommend are Solgar's Advanced Acidophilus 40+ and the prebiotic, Bimuno.

8) Flexibility: Stretching exercises to maintain or improve the flexibility of muscles, tendons and joints is of paramount

importance, especially before intense resistance training. (see DVD)

9) Intense short interval training e.g. Tabata   Rather than doing long, drawn out aerobic sessions, intense intervals has been shown to increase oxygen uptake and capillary network to muscles without reducing muscle size and strength. When done 3 x weekly, massive hikes in aerobic/anaerobic fitness will ensue.

10) Periodisation: It is important to plan your workouts to allow for full recovery of both the muscles and tendons. It may be that a 3 day split routine is enough to allow this. Something like Monday: chest/triceps/ shoulders, Tuesday: legs, Thursday: Back, Biceps, Abs. This gives enough days rest to recover. This will allow maximum intensity to be used on each workout without fear of overtraining. Use the following plan:

Week 1) ECCENTRIC

Week 2) OXIDATIVE

Week 3) GLYCOLYTIC

Week 4) ECCENTRIC

Repeat this cycle 2 or 3 times, then take a whole week off resistance work. Eccentric working sets should be no more than 6 reps and 10 seconds for each rep. If time under tension goes over 60 secs ie more than 6 reps,then up the weight a fraction for next time. Oxidative reps are over 10 and no more than 15, adjusting the weight as needed. Glycolytic is 6-8 reps lasting 30 secs per set.

11) Andropause: As we age, our release of testosterone diminishes, increased levels of SHBG pulls usable testosterone from the blood and binds it up , so it cannot pass its message on at the receptor sites. Symptoms are: low energy, increased fat mass, lower muscle mass, low self-esteem, low libido, erectile dysfunction, depression. It can also lead to osteopenia or osteoporosis and cardiac problems. Initial treatment is intensive

resistance training, Vit D3 and zinc supplementation. If after 6 months, levels of FSH, LH and testosterone are still not rising, then an endocrinologist should be sought for possible HRT therapy. Regular blood tests should also check Homocysteine and Haematocrit levels.

Supplements to be considered are : Serrapeptase, Nattokinase, Solgar's Homocysteine regulator and enteric coated Aspirin 75mg.

12) Somatopause: From age 30 onwards, your GH and IGF-1 natural levels deplete rapidly. Also the pulsatile release of GH during the day as a response from exercise and at night during sleep are reduced in intensity. Symptoms are loss of muscle mass, gains in fat mass, loss of elastin in skin (more wrinkles), lower energy and general wellbeing, loss of bone density, increase in total cholesterol.

Treatment is initially carefully scheduling your intense weights and intense aerobics along with good sleep patterns. Taking L-Arginine, preferably in a good pharmaceutical grade with the correct synergists (ProArgi9+). Retest IGF-1 and IGF-BP3 levels after 6 months. If still low, consider either Sermorelin or GH replacement therapy from an endocrinologist or reputable clinic.

13) Haemodynamics: Maintenance of blood flow to the tissues is of paramount importance to maximise both performance and recovery. In order to minimise the stress response affecting haemodynamics, we recommend monthly massage and fascial release sessions for the soft-tissues and 2 or 3 monthly sessions for the hard tissues using manipulation and acupuncture techniques.

For those people suffering nocturnal or daytime cramping following intense workouts try increasing calcium/magnesium and include niacin to help dilate blood vessel and restore balance in the muscles.

14) The Prostate Gland: BPH (Benign Prostatic Hypertrophy) occurs in older men over 50 years. It seems to have a tentative link to those who took anabolic steroids in the past, probably due to high levels of DHT. It most cases, it does not progress to cancer, but it can cause urinary problems.It may be controlled by the drug, Finasteride or naturally by long term use of Saw Palmetto. PSA is not a good indicator of Prostate Cancer. To prevent unnecessary biopsies being taken, a PCA 3 test or Urine Exosome Assay Gene Assay test can be done.

CONCLUSIONS

So there you have it! I have tried to be as accurate scientifically with the current level of knowledge to provide everything you need in this book to create the best, healthy physique possible! All the tools you need are here to maximise your potential. I have tried to cut through all the Hype and confusion you see with conflicting information on the internet and in Health and Fitness magazines. Be aware that often people are trying to sell a product or push a fad. Be prepared to challenge everything and be aware that even research can be flawed! Very often interested parties will steer research to reach their own required conclusions! If you wish to check things out Scientifically, don't just read one article on a subject, read many and make sure it is peer reviewed before you even consider accepting it as fact! This method will allow you to rise above the rest and be your own man (or woman). Don't be a 'sheep' following blindly some so-called Guru simply because he has a strong personality or even physique! Be aware that many bodybuilders with freaky physiques aren't always following these methods in this book. Many who have superior genetics will achieve an amazing physique following any type of resistance program. All I can tell you is that if you want to achieve YOUR maximum potential, then follow these principles. I remember Dorian saying to another amazing genetically gifted Bodybuilder (who had even better genetics than Dorian), 'You will never be Mr Olympia (i.e. never beat him) unless you put my head on your body'. So even a genetically gifted bodybuilder would never reach his potential unless he fully applied himself to these principles.

Very best wishes and enjoy challenging your body to reach greater heights,

Stuart

An instructional DVD
accompanies this book

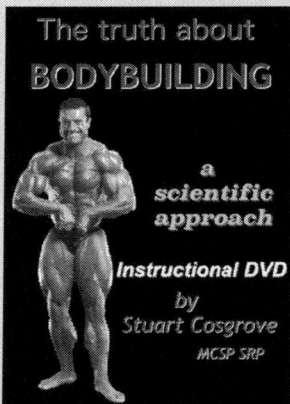

The truth about
BODYBUILDING

a
scientific
approach

Instructional DVD
by
Stuart Cosgrove
MCSP SRP

To order this DVD
please either send
by post or scan this
page and email using
the voucher code
below. This will prove
you own a copy of the
book

PRICE £12-99 inc postage

email to: cosgrovesphysio@btconnect.com
Please fill in all details below:

NAME:
ADDRESS:

POSTCODE:
CREDIT CARD DETAILS:
Card number:
Name on card:
Valid from: **To:**
3 Digit security code:

voucher code   J14k78

234

REFERENCES

CHAPTER 1
Henry Gray-Gray's Anatomy, Foss ML and Keteyian SJ -Fox's Physiological basis for exercise and sport (1998) Rasmussen RB and Philips SM - Contractile and Nutritional Regulation of Human Muscle Growth (2003), Herbert A Devries- Physiology of Exercise (1984), McArdle,Katch,Katch- Exercise physiology (2001)

CHAPTER 2
Herbert A devries-Physiology of Exercise(1984), McArdle,Katch,Katch -Exercise Physiology (2001), Costill DL et al - Skeletal muscle enzymes and fibre composition in female track athletes, jornal of applied physiology (1976), Dahmane R et al - Spatial fibre type distribution in normal muscle,journal of biomechanics (2005), Edgerton VR et al - muscle fibre type poulations in human leg muscles (1975), Fry AC et al - Muscle fibre charactreristics of competitive powerlifters, Journal of Strength and conditioning research (2003), Johnson M et al - Data on distribution of fibre types in 36 human muscles an autopsy study,Journal of neurological sciences (1973), Ogborn D et al -The role of fibre types in Hypertrophy-Implications for loading strategies (2014), Scott W et al- Human muscle fibre type classifications (2001)

CHAPTER 3
Charge SBP and Rudnicki MA - Cellular and molecular regulation of muscle regeneration, physiological reviews volume 84 (2004), Rasmussen RB and Phillips SM - Contractile and nutritional regulation of human muscle growth (2003), Joulia-Ekaza D,Cabello G - The myostatin gene -physiologacal and pharmacological relevance (2007), Tsuchida K - Targetting myostatin for therapies against muscle wasting diseases, Kambadur R et al -mutations in myostatin in double muscled belgian blue and piedmontese cattle (1997), Peter Mitchell - cryoflow revolutionising physical therapy(2004) , Armal MA et al,- Protein pulse feeding improves protein retention in elderly women, Journal of Clinical Nutrition (1999), Boirie Y et al -

235

Slow and fast dietary proteins differently modulate postprandial protein accretion (1997), Borsheim E et al -Essential amino acids and muscle protein recovery from resistance exercise, Anderson L.L et al - The effects of resistance training combined with timed ingestion of protein on muscle fibre size and strength (2005), Costill DL et al - Adaptations in skeleltal muscle following strength training ,Journal of applied physiology (1979), McCall GE et al - Muscle fibre hypertrophy,hyperplasia and capillary density on college men after resistance training, Journal of applied physiology, Goldspink DF et al - Muscle growth in response to mechanical stimuli (1995), McMahon G et al - Muscular adaptations and IGF 1 responses to resistance training are stretch mediated (2014),D'Antona G et al - Skeletal muscle hypertrophy and structure and function of skeletal muscle fibres in male bodybuilders ,Journal of physiology (2006), Deschenes MR and Kraemer WJ, -Performance and physiologic adaptations to resistance training American journal of physical medicine (2002).

CHAPTER 4

Peter Mitchell- Cryoflow Revolutionising Physical therapy (2004), Hakkinen K et al - Neuromuscular adaptations during concurrent strength and endurance training versus strength training ,European journal of applied physiology (2003) , Bishop D et al - The effects of strength training on endurance performance and muscle characteristics (1999). Herbert A Devries-Physiology of exercise (1984), Clark RA et al - The influence of variable range of motion on neuromuscular performance and control of external loads- J strength cond res (2011), McArdle WD et al - Exercise physiology (2001).

CHAPTER 5

Menno Henselmans -Partial v Full Reps (2015) , Legionathletics.com occlusiontraining, Gaines C - Yours in perfect manhood-Charles Atlas (1982), Ellington Darden phD - The Bodyfat breakthrough (2014) , Craig Cecil - Bodybuilding from Heavy Duty to Superslow (2012), Gary Bannister - If you like Exercise,chances are your doing it wrong (2013), Jones A - Nautilus Training Principles Bulletins (1971) , Brian D Johnston - Higher Intelligence Training (2005),.Simoneau J A   et al-

Isokinetic Strength training Protocols: Do they induce skeletal muscle fibre Hypertrophy? (1988), E.F.Coyle et al - Specificity of power improvements through slow and fast isokinetic training,Journal of applied physiology (1981), Jackson CGR et al - Skeletal muscle fibre area alterations in two opposing modes of resistance training in the same individual, European journal of Applied physiology (1990),Schlumberger A et al: Different effects on human muscle heavy chain isoform expression stength v combination training,Journal of Applied Physiology(2003), Netreba A et al Responses of Knee extensor muscles to leg press training of various types (2013)Schoenfeld BJ et al -Muscular adaptations in low v high resistance training programs

CHAPTER 6

Ellington Darden phD- The bodyfat breakthrough (2014) , Per A Tesch phD - Target Bodybuilding (1999), Craig Cecil, Bodybuilding from Heavy Duty to Superslow (2012), Craig Bannister-If you like Exercise,chances are your doing it wrong (2013), Jones A, Nautilus training principles bulletins (1971), Brian D Johnston-Higher Intelligence Training (2005), Campos GE et al- Muscular adaptations in response to three different resistance training regimes , European Journal of applied Physiology (2002), Carroll TJ et al- Resistance training frequency ,European Journal of applied physiology (1998), Evangelidis PE et al - The functional significance of Hamstrings composition-Is it really a fast muscle group , Scandinavian Journal of medicine and science in sports (2016), Fry AC et al- Muscle fibre composition of competitive powerlifters, Journal of strength and conditioning research (2003), Fry AC- The Role of resistance training intensity on muscle fibre adaptations , Sports medicine (2004), Hather BM et al - The influence of eccentric actions on skeletal muscle adaptations to resistance training (1991), Jackson CGR et al - Skeletal muscle fibre area alterations in two opposing modes of resistance training in the same individual , European Journal of applied physiology(1990), Ogborn D and Schoenfeld BJ - The role of fibre types in Muscle hypertrophy: Implications for loading strategies, Strength and conditioning journal (2014), Paddon-Jones D et al - Adaptation to chronic eccentric exercise in humans (2001), Schoenfeld BJ et al -

Muscular adaptations in low versus high load resistance training, European journal of sports science (2014), Raue U et al - Effects of short term concentric v eccentric resistance training on a single muscle fibre MHC distribution in humans, International journal of sports medicine (2005), Schuenke MD et al - Early phase muscular adaptations in response to slow speed versus traditional resistance training regimens , European journal of applied physiology (2012), Goldspink DF - Muscle growth in response to mechanical stimuli , Am J Physiology (1995), Goldspink GJ - Changes in muscle mass and phenotype and the expression of autocrine and systemic growth factors in response to stretch and overload (1999), Drinkwater EJ et al - Effects of changing from full range of motion to partial range on squat kinetics-Journal of strength and conditioning research (2012), Bazyler CD et al - The efficacy of incorporating partial squats in maximal strength training J strength cond res (2014), Gentil P et al - Time under Tension and Blood lactate response during 4 different Resistance Training methods-J of Physiological Anthropology (2006).

CHAPTER 7
Ellington Darden phD - The Bodyfat breakthrough (2014), Per A Tesch PhD - Target Bodybuilding (1999), Fry AC - The role of exercise intensity on muscle fibre adaptations, Sports medicine (2004), Hather BM et al - The influence of eccentric contractions on skeletal muscle adaptations to resistance training (1991), Jones N et al - A genetic based algorithm for personalized resistance training, Biology of sport (2016), Paddon-Jones D et al - Adaptation to chronic eccentric exercise in humans- the influence of contraction velocity, E.J Applied physiology (2001), Putman CT et al - Effects of strength,endurance and combined training on myosin heavy chain content and fibre type distribution in humans, E.J. applied physiology (2004), Raue U et al - Effects of short term concentric v eccentric loading on a single muscle fibre MHC distribution in humans, I.J sports medicine (2005)

CHAPTER 8
Rasmussen RB and Phillips SM - Contractile and nutritional regulation of human muscle growth (2003), Dr Millward J et al -

238

Protein quality assaessment , American journal of clinical nutrition (2008), Stephen van Vliet et al - The skeletal muscle Anabolic response to animal v plant protein consumption , J of Nutrition (2015), expert-nutrition.com - Protein quality-why some proteins are better than others (2018), Clarkson P and Thompson H - Antioxidants-What role do they play in physical activity and health? , American journal for clinical nutrition (2000), Kanter M - Free radicals, exercise and antioxidant supplementation (1998), Karlsson J - Antioxidants and exercise (1997), Peter Mitchell - Revolutionising physical therapy (2004), Threlkeld A - The effects of manual therapy on connective tissue , Cantu R and Grodin A - Myofascial manipulation (1992), Leon Chaitlow- masterclass in palpation and the body fascia(1999), Fields GB - The collagen triple helix connective tissue research (1995), Goldspink GJ et al - Changes in muscle fibre type, muscle mass and IGF 1 expression in rabbit skeletal muscle subject to stretch (1997), Dattilo M et al - Sleep and muscle recovery.

CHAPTER 9
Lennard Funk-Shoulderdoc.co.uk 2019, Maitlands Spinal manipulation(8th edition) 2005, Peter Ueblacker et al-Muscle Injuries in Sports (2010) , Pedrelli A, Stecco C, Day JA - Treating Patellar Tendinopathy with Fascial Manipulation (2009), Stecco C, Day JA - The Fascial Manipulation Technique and its Biomechanical Model, A guide to the Human Fascial System ,National library of Medicine De Puy Synthes Companies - Understanding Conditions physiopedia.com and Headache Therapy.org, Threlkeld A, The effects of Manual Therapy on connective tissue, Cantu R, Grodin A - Myofascial manipulation (1992), Leon Chaitlow - Masterclass in palpation and the body fascia (1999), Fields GB - The Collagen triple Helix Connective tissue research.

CHAPTER 10
Rodriguez NR et al - Nutrition and athletic performance-Medicine and science in sports and exercise (2009), Lachlan Mitchell et al - Do bodybuilders use evidence based nutrition strategies to manipulate physique (2017), NCSA Kinetic select and Lowery L phD - Dietary fat and performance (2017),

Clarkson P and Thompson H - Antioxidants-what role do they play in physical activity and health? -American society for clinical nutrition (2000), Kanter M - Free radicals, exercise and antioxidant supplementation (1998), Karlsson J - Antioxidants and exercise-Human kinetics (1997), Dr Michael Kendrick - The great Cholesterol Con (2007), Berberine, Creatine, citrulline, beta-alanine all peer reviewed research by examine.com, Arnal MA et al - Protein pulse feeding improves protein retention in elderly women - Am journal of clin nutrition, Boirie Y et al - Slow and fast dietary proteins differently modulate postprandial protein accretion (1997), Borsheim E at al - Essential amino acids and muscle protein recovery from resistance exercise - Am J Physiol Endocrinol Metab (2002), Anderson LL et al - The effect of resistance training combined with timed ingestion of protein on muscle fibre size and strength (2005).

CHAPTER 11
World Anabolic review-P Grunding and M Bachmann (1997), Anabolics 2000, Joseph King - the big book of steroids (2016), Joulia-Ekaza D, cabello G - The myostatin gene-physiology and pharmacological relevance (2007), Tsuchida K (2008), Targetting myostatin for therapies against muscle wasting diseases, Ken KY Ho - Growth Hormone- Endocrinology and metabolism clinics of north america (2007), Dr Malcolm Kendrick - The Great Cholesterol Con (2007), Berberine, creatine,citrulline, Beta-alanine - peer reviewed research by examine.com (2019), Druzhevskaya AM et al - Association of the ACTN3 gene polymorphism with power athlete status in Russians-J of Applied physiology (2008), Goldspink G et al - Mechano growth factor E peptide derived from IGF 1 activates human muscle cells and induces an increase in their fusion potential at different ages (2017), Kraemer WJ et al - Compatibility of high intensity strength and endurance training on hormonal and skeletal muscle adaptations- J of applied physiology (1995), Ma F et al - The association of sport performance with ACE and ACTN3 genetic polymorphisms: a systematic review and meta-analysis (2013), Papadimitriou ID et al - The ACTN3 gene in elite Greek track and field athletes -Int J of sports medicine (2008), Roth SM et al - The ACTN3 R577X nonsense allele is under-represented in elite level

240

strength athletes- Europ J of Human Genetics (2008), Goldspink G - Changes in muscle mass and phenotype and the expression of autocrine and systemic growth factors by muscle in response to stretch and overload (1999), McMahon et al - Muscular adaptations and IGF 1 responses to resistance training are stretch mediated (2014), Vanhee C et al - Analysis of illegal peptide biopharmaceuticals frequently encountered by controlling agencies (2015), Goldspink G - research on mechano growth factor : its potential for optimising physical training as well as misuse in doping-B.J. Sports med (2005), Mehrpour M et al - Effects of low intensity Continuous ultrasound on Hemotological parameters of Rats -J Biomed Phys Eng (2016), Robbins RC et al - Ingestion of Grapefruit lowers haematocrits in human subjects- Int J of Vitamin nutrition(1988), Pro Argi 9+ Human clinical studies at High Desert heart Institute by Dr Siva Arunasdam.(2019).

CHAPTER 12

Ken KY Ho _ Growth Hormone- The endocrinology and metabolism clinics of North America (2007), sermorelin structure- Pub Chem database(2019), Sermorelin -Empower pharmacy (2018), Is Somatopause an Indication for Growth hormone replacement- Savine R,Sonksen PH - J endocrinology (1999),Benbassat CA et al - Circulationg levels of IGF 1 and 3 in Aging men - J of clinical endocrinology and metabolism, Dattilo M et al - Sleep and muscle recovery (2011), Walker RF - Sermorelin: A better approach to management of adult onset GH insuficiency? (2006), Without a blind amino acid rider, oral L-arginine is unsafe in humans-Journal of American Medical association/John Hopkins university (2003), Dr Malcolm Kendrick - The Great Cholesterol Con (2007), Arnal MA - Protein Pulse feeding improves protein retention in elderly women -Am J Clin Nutr (1999), Anianson A and Gustafsson E - Physical training in elderly men with special reference to quadriceps muscle strength and morphology- Clinical physiology (1981),Charette SL et al - Muscle Hypertrophy response to resistance training in older women-J of App Physiology (1991), Churchward- Venne TA et al - There are no nonresponders to resistance type exercise training in older men and women (2015), Frontera WR et al - Skeletal Muscle fibre quality in older men

241

and women- Am j of Physiology (2000), Hakkinen K et al - Changes in EMG activity , muscle fibre force characteristics during heavy resistance training in middle aged and older men and women (2001),Goldspink G et al - Mechano growth factor E peptide derived from IGF 1 activates human muscle cells and induces an increase in their fusion potential at different ages (2017), Karavirta L et al - Effects of combined endurance and strength training on muscle strength , power and hypertrophy in 40-67 year old men- Scandinavian J of Med and science in Sports (2011), Kosek DJ et al - Efficacy of 3 days/week resistance training on myofibre hypertrophy and myogenic mechanisms in young v older adults- J of App physiology (2006), McGuigan MR et al - Resistance training in patients with Peripheral artery disease effects on muscle myoforms,fibre type distributionand capillary supply to skeletal muscle -The J of Gerontology series A (2001), Malisoux L et al - Calcium sensitivity of single fibre human muscle following plyometric training-Medicine and science in sports and exercise (2006), Nygaard E and Sanchez J- Intramuscular variation of fibre types in the biceps and vastus lateralis of elderly men - The anatomical record (1982), PyKa G et al - Muscle strength and fibre adaptations to a year long resistance program in elderly men and women-J of Gerontology (1994), Robbins RC et al - Ingestion of Grapefruit lowers haematocrits in human subjects - Int J of Vitamins nutrition (1988), Mehrpour M et al - Effects of low intensity ultrasound on Hematological Parameters on Rats - J Biomed Phys Eng (2016), ProArgi 9+ helps prevent Kidney failure and many other podcasts on You tube by Dr Joseph Prendergast from Sacramento Heart Centre, ProArgi 9+ can do what L-Arginine cannot do on its own- Hughes centre for research(2019), Li JV et al - Biology of the Microbiome-Gastroenterology Clinics of North America(2017), Microbiome and diet -Dept of surgery and cancer ,Imperial college of London (2019), Microbiome - University of Southampton Study (2019). Multiple podcasts and seminars by Dr Michael Hamblin on the Benefits of Red Light therapy, LDL Cholesterol does not cause cardiovascular disease- a comprehensive review of the current literature- Ravnskov U et al -Expert review of Clinical Pharmacology (2018), Sommer AP and Zhu D - Green tea and Red light- a powerful duo in skin rejuvenation.

Printed in Poland
by Amazon Fulfillment
Poland Sp. z o.o., Wrocław